KICKING THE DIET MINDSET

THE ULTIMATE GUIDE TO STOP BINGE EATING AND START EATING INTUITIVELY

GABRIELLE TOWNSEND

SILK PUBLISHING

CONTENTS

Foreword	v
Introduction	ix
1. What Is Intuitive Eating?	1
2. Identifying The Problem	16
3. Hunger Is The Enemy	34
4. It's All In Your Head!	42
5. Exercise - The Way to Look and Feel Better	49
6. How Do I Actually Eat Intuitively?	64
7. My 5 Step Process To Success	73
8. Stop Blaming Yourself	79
9. Surround Yourself With the Right Environment	95
10. Seeking Help and Finding a Community	103
Afterword	109
References	117

FOREWORD

If you have a history of constantly being drawn to a new diet or gimmick to help you lose those unwanted pounds and you seem to be getting nowhere slowly, and you've come to the point where you simply don't know who to trust anymore because there are too many conflicting dieting concepts out there—this book is especially for you.

Here you will learn how to take a complete break from what you've been brainwashed into believing: that to be loved by someone, or accepted by society, you need to fit into this size, you need to be this shape, or you need to belong to a community of dieters.

If you're feeling overwhelmed and confused by all the conflicting messages and diets available out there, you've found a solution. Your confusion is natural because there are so many conflicting messages and diets out there. Virtually everywhere you look there's some new miracle cure popping up on your Facebook feed. It's no wonder that the diet industry is thriving: it's a multi-billion-dollar industry after all.

By now, you're probably tired of asking yourself which of the diets out there is right for your age, shape, height, personal preference, blood type, and even your culture? After all, you've probably tried a few and failed more often than not. Many of the diets available start off promising and then all of a sudden you notice the pounds creeping back on, plus a little extra for good measure.

I'm here to burst the dieting bubble and to let you know that none of them are doing you any good at all! Yep, you heard me—the best diet you can be on right now is NO DIET! And no, I'm not the first person to come up with this theory. As a matter of fact, this belief has been kicking around since the 1970s, with it finally being given the official label of "intuitive eating" for the first time in 1995.

What makes this different from every other diet out there? While it's a relatively simple concept, many find it more difficult to learn and apply to their lives daily. Intuitive eating is based on the simple philosophy of eating when you are hungry and stopping when your body is feeling satisfied. It's moving away from starving yourself for extended periods between meals like you would do for example during intermittent fasting.

Another main objective of intuitive eating is to build an effective barrier against binge eating. Intuitive eating is actually the complete opposite of a diet. There's no calorie counting or restriction involved. Because it's designed this way you won't suffer from craving all the goodies on the 'bad food list.' As a matter of fact, there is no good or bad food list with intuitive eating.

FOREWORD

Intuitive eating takes time to learn and practice. It means learning to listen to what your body is telling you, rather than allowing your mind to be in control. Intuitive eating encourages you to eat anything that you want and learning to accept your body image. Learning to love who you are and what you look like. This acceptance is the key to living a life that's happier and more fulfilled, irrespective of what you look like.

In the pages that follow we'll discuss ways to introduce intuitive eating into your life so you can regain control over your lifestyle and never have to diet again.

It will teach you that you can still enjoy the foods you want to eat in moderation without feeling guilty about what you're putting into your mouth. It replaces the constant fear of not being able to fit into your favorite pair of jeans with the freedom to love yourself for who you are, as you are!

© **Copyright 2020 - All rights reserved.**

The content contained within this book may not be reproduced, duplicated or transmitted without direct written permission from the author or the publisher.

Under no circumstances will any blame or legal responsibility be held against the publisher, or author, for any damages, reparation, or monetary loss due to the information contained within this book, either directly or indirectly.

Legal Notice:

This book is copyright protected. It is only for personal use. You cannot amend, distribute, sell, use, quote or paraphrase any part, or the content within this book, without the consent of the author or publisher.

Disclaimer Notice:

Please note the information contained within this document is for educational and entertainment purposes only. All effort has been executed to present accurate, up to date, reliable, complete information. No warranties of any kind are declared or implied. Readers acknowledge that the author is not engaged in the rendering of legal, financial, medical or professional advice. The content within this book has been derived from various sources. Please consult a licensed professional before attempting any techniques outlined in this book.

By reading this document, the reader agrees that under no circumstances is the author responsible for any losses, direct or indirect, that are incurred as a result of the use of the information contained within this document, including, but not limited to, errors, omissions, or inaccuracies.

INTRODUCTION

"Diets, like clothes, should be tailored to you."

— JOAN RIVERS

Do you suffer from mood swings resulting in feelings of guilt, depression and anxiety constantly because of your addiction to a fad, weight loss gimmick, or diet? Are you one of those shoppers who counts calories on every item before adding it to your cart? This is often happening on a subconscious level and because you've been doing it for so many years, you don't even realize that you're doing it anymore.

Do you feel extreme anxiety and remorse when you've enjoyed a night out with your friends or that special someone, knowing that you've overindulged? Are these sorrowful sentiments likely to linger with you longer than you'd like them to? Or do you try and figure out what your next step is going to be to get rid of the additional calories you've carelessly overindulged in? Are your eating decisions putting you on a "permanent guilt trip" rather than allowing you to enjoy the important things you want and deserve from life?

If you had to identify the category that you fall within, would you admit to being addicted to a diet? There are so many individuals simply going through the motions of life—one with little to no joy because they constantly feel desperately unhappy about what they look like. They don't like the way their clothes fit, and they are permanently uncomfortable about their weight. For these individuals, picking up 500g is too much to deal with, let alone packing on a couple of extra pounds for no reason.

Do you shudder every time you need to visit a medical professional for a routine check-up and they ask you to climb on a weight scale? You're almost waiting for it to show an 'error' reading because it can't handle your weight!

Does the very thought of holidays or special celebrations leave you feeling depressed because you know that it's going to result in any weight you've managed to lose piling right back on again? Is your anxiety worsened by all the traditional 'food-based' holidays like Thanksgiving, Easter, Christmas, Mother's Day, Father's Day, weddings and anniversaries, not to mention any birthdays in between?

Is walking past your local bakery simply too tempting to pass up the chance for fresh bagels or croissants? Can you tie some of your physical anxiety to food? Do you turn to food whenever you're bored or emotional? Or has that extra helping of whatever you ate at dinner left you feeling bloated, uncomfortable and unable to sleep?

If you can relate to any of the above emotions or expe-

INTRODUCTION

riences, this book may just be what you need to regain some of the control over your life. While you may not realize it at this moment, you actually have more control and say in your association with food than you are willing to admit to.

We'd all like to be thin... I mean, who can blame you for feeling this way when everywhere you look, 90 lbs. models adorn glossy magazines, movies, advertisements, and even Instagram. Every woman wants to be the "perfect" size with ideal measurements to match, but let's get real for a moment: we are all unique and different. These differences should be accepted and celebrated rather than send you on a lifelong guilt-trip due to the body type you were born with.

Because of this ideology that's placed on girls from a young age, many women begin dieting from the time they're a teenager and things kind of literally go "pear-shape" from there on out. Yo-yo dieting becomes the norm, each time resulting in more and more weight returning than before. For some, the perfect body only begins to disappear once children arrive! After the first child, things usually get back to normal fairly quickly. By baby number 2 it can become a bit harder. The weight is harder to get off and keep off, especially that bulge directly around the midriff that closely resembles a flotation device. No amount of dieting seems to make even the slightest dent in getting rid of this excess weight that you're constantly carrying around with you wherever you go.

Between the sleepless nights tending to a newborn baby and possibly chasing after another toddler, you'd think that all the excess weight would just melt away magically. Unfortunately, if you happened to undergo a cesarean section, your chances of getting rid of that spare weight around your waistline make finding a unicorn in your garden to be a more realistic possibility.

Because you're exhausted and emotional, you turn to your comfort food of choice, whatever this may be (and chances are, it's nothing healthy like carrot sticks or a fruit smoothie). It probably resembles something with loads of calories, that you absolutely know you're going to regret in the morning, or whenever you next step on the scale.

Finding the time for an exercise regime is virtually impossible, especially if you need to catch up on your own nap time by synchronizing it with baby for the first few weeks and months.

No matter how old you are, once the dieting merry-go-round begins, it's more and more difficult to get off the longer you remain on it. While diets themselves are restrictive in terms of what you can or can't eat, the effects on your mental health begin to take their toll. Every time you happen to crave that special treat and give in to temptation and indulge, you feel guilty about it and this leads to anxiety, which could, in turn, lead to depression.

In an article written by (Sauer, 2018), she admitted… "I feel anxious about my body and anxious about what I eat. I often find myself overeating when presented with "off-limits" foods and feeling guilty about it far too often."

There's no miracle cure and "one-size-fits-all" when it comes to dieting—why? Because each of us is totally different and unique. We each have different DNA and blood types, our body types are different and for some,

INTRODUCTION

metabolism comes into play. The thyroid can wreak havoc on the entire system making weight loss an impossibility—yet we all still desire the perfect body to make us feel good about ourselves. We feel as though if we have the perfect body all will be right in the world.

Intuitive eating gives us the formula and means to develop another way of life. It deals with not only your physical side but your mental and emotional side as well. It's about learning to listen to your body when making decisions about what you plan on putting into it in terms of what you eat. Listening to your body initially can be tricky and you're bound to have a number of bumps in the road as you begin this exciting new journey off the dieting-merry-go-round!

The main thing with intuitive eating is to trash your thoughts of ever dieting again. It's getting rid of all your previously attempted diets that simply made you more frustrated daily. It's kicking out the Keto recipes, archiving your ancient Atkins diet book, banishing the "Blood Type" diet and any other failed fad your body has never quite responded to. From taking pills that are supposed to magically dissolve fatty deposits around your body to intermittent fasting routines, many of you would have possibly tried a number of these only to have all the weight creep back the moment you stopped.

For those with underlying health issues such as diabetes, heart, lung or back problems that prevent them from participating in the high-intensity exercise programs needed to support each of these diets, there's simply no hope or light at the end of the tunnel. All that this results in is leaving you feeling miserable and dejected.

Personally, I have struggled with the mentality of diets, often losing weight only to gain it all back again, or going all out and destroying any momentum I may have gained by rigidly sticking with the diet by binge eating. I'm the first to admit that dieting for me simply doesn't work and I had to find a new approach to discovering how to eat what I want when I want while being mindful of not only my health but my body as well.

The natural benefit to approaching intuitive eating is discovering joy in your life, rather than constantly being on edge, counting carbs or calories, or cringing every time you walk past a store that sells food that's on your "do not touch" list.

It's actually being able to keep the weight off, instead of an endless yo-yo weight on, weight off effect. It's being confident and comfortable getting on your bathroom scale without worrying about what the numbers say!

Intuitive eating allows me to enjoy those foods that I want when I want them by learning to listen to what my body is telling me.

My main reason for writing *Kicking the Diet Mindset* is that I realized I am the best person—the only person—who can actually make these choices for me. I realized that following every new crazy diet was not the solution that I was looking for, or what was best for me in the long run. I also wanted to share what I have learned about this completely new way of looking at your personal relationship with food with others who may, like I was, totally frustrated with being bombarded constantly with this diet, shake or pill!

With my help and expertise, by following the tips and suggestions in *Kicking the Diet Mindset,* you will be fully

INTRODUCTION

equipped to discover and deal with your body image. Whether you are happy with your body right now or not, it's important to get there properly with all the facts at your disposal.

Are you currently keen on trying out yet another diet? Go ahead, but let's look at your history to date, as well as the history of others. If you genuinely want to remain healthy, physically and mentally throughout life it's going to come from knowing yourself and your limits and learning to eat intuitively.

No human is meant to be dieting for 80-plus years: whether healthy or not, it's been proven that people only have a certain capacity for deprivation before they break.

What if you never have to break? What if eating good food and splurging sometimes can actually be fun?

Don't waste another year of your life binge eating and then punishing yourself mentally and emotionally for it.

Every chapter in this book is structured in a way that will provide you with actionable steps that can help you choose what is truly best for your body in both the short and long term. Stop being distracted by every new trend, tool, course or diet (all this is achieving is presenting you with "Shiny Object Syndrome"). Identify what the problem is and fix it immediately.

If you follow the methods outlined in this book, it is very likely that you will never struggle with clarity around dieting again.

1

WHAT IS INTUITIVE EATING?

"As you go through your day, try to look at food differently. Look at how it works for your body: nourishing it, fueling, and allowing pleasure. Notice how food feels friendly when you eat intuitively, if food is there for you as a friend. Can you feel the difference?

— *FOOD: FRIEND AND FUEL? – STAY ATTUNED*

INTRODUCTION TO WHAT INTUITIVE EATING IS

Understanding what intuitive eating is takes us back to how we behaved as children. It's a way of eating that we've forgotten as we moved into adulthood. Instead of drinking a bottle until we were full or eating what was on our plate until we were full, then returning to play, we've become like robots in our eating habits.

Rather than stopping, we eat until the plate is empty,

no matter how big it is, and too often we've piled way too much on the plate in the first place. Intuitive eating promotes a healthy outlook towards the food that we eat and prevent us from over-indulging. The theory behind it is to eat when you are hungry, rather than when you're absolutely ravenous, and to stop eating when you are feeling content or comfortable, rather than bloated due to overeating.

Its name indicates that you should follow your own "intuition" regarding your need for food and feeling satisfied. While this is implied, there are not many individuals who know where this invisible line begins or ends. Imagine that you could measure your hunger on a scale or measuring stick, where zero is the point where you are absolutely starving/ravenous for your next morsel of food, and 10 is the point where you are about to explode because you're feeling totally stuffed (and you know you're going to regret it in the morning)! The scale has different points that measure variations of hunger or being satisfied.

The idea behind intuitive eating is to eat when you are hungry and stop when you are content, or comfortable. Realistically, it's probably ranging between 2 and 7 or 8 on the scale depending on your current size and body type (and yes, your body type can affect all of this). It could also be influenced by other medical factors which we'll cover a bit further on.

Many people don't know how to measure this for themselves and have forgotten these cues that the body gives off, letting the brain know when it needs to be fed and when it's had enough. This is what intuitive eating is going to teach you—how to listen to that inner voice more closely so that you can begin living a life free of food guilt forever (or as close to it as possible)!

Following an intuitive eating plan is literally having to learn how to eat correctly all over again (regardless of your current age).

Intuitive eating is more than just learning when to start and stop eating to stay alive—it's also about accepting your body image and learning to love yourself for who you are. This is probably going to be the most challenging part of this journey, but once you have learned how to accept who you are, you will become happier, feel more fulfilled, and live a life that's more joyous than ever before.

WHAT INTUITIVE EATING ISN'T

It's not another new-age diet or fad to follow. It's a way of life that once adopted will change your outlook on life forever. In fact, intuitive eating has been around since the 1970s and can hardly be called ground-breaking. What is currently trending though is that there is more research and scientific data being gathered and presented in support of intuitive eating.

It's not going to break your bank balance—there are no fancy tablets, meal plans, shakes, smoothies, meetings or other gimmicks that you need to buy to get started (and then be hooked on for an indefinite period).

You get to decide for yourself what foods you'd like to eat, rather than being given a strict dietary routine that can become totally boring after following it religiously for the first week or so.

With intuitive eating, there's no need to count out

calories or measure how many potatoes you're allowed per day. Intuitive eating is completely opposite to a diet. You're actually encouraged to eat the foods that you want, rather than a miserable lettuce leaf and a few carrot sticks as your evening meal!

There is a difference between mindful eating and intuitive eating—although they are similar, they are also different.

THE HISTORY OF INTUITIVE EATING

Evelyn Tribole and Elyse Resch, two well-known and respected dieticians and obesity experts, first wrote *Intuitive Eating: A Revolutionary Program that Works* in 1995 to share their ideas on the philosophy of getting off of diets completely by redefining your relationship with food. They included step-by-step methods that could be used to break habits of emotional eating which we could probably refer to as our comfort food, or binge-eating preferences today. Many saw this book as a revolutionary new way to approach how we eat, although there had already been quite a bit of work on the topic, done by Susie Orbach (1978), who published "Fat is a Feminist Issue," and even Geneen Roth (1982) who wrote about emotional eating habits. All these women were classified as early pioneers in this research and while the term "Intuitive Eating" was only coined in 1995, there were weight management programs founded by Thelma Wayler (1973) known as Green Mountain at Fox Run, which was based in Vermont.

Since then, there have been many more intensive research studies to support intuitive eating, and which we will cover below, but the main emphasis of the entire program was built on the premise that conventional diets don't work and that important changes in personal care are necessary for long-term health.

RESEARCH ON INTUITIVE EATING

In this section we are going to focus on research that has been done since this revolutionary way of eating was discovered—and since the call to "ban the diet completely" was expressed.

The interesting part of this process is that none of these authors or those looking to implement the intuitive eating plan were gym enthusiasts or entrepreneurs, promoting their latest "secret weapon against beating the bulge"; instead, they were all reputable dieticians who had years of experience to back up their theories and methodologies.

We are going to devote the rest of this chapter to discussing some of the studies done since the early days of Evelyn Tribole and Elyse Resch (1995) first putting pen to paper and publishing their book which proved to be the catalyst and game changer on intuitive eating. Up until this point, it hadn't even been given a name. The very first time the words "intuitive eating" were ever recorded and used to name this way of eating was by Tribole and Resch in 1995.

Let's look at a study conducted in a number of universities located in New Zealand, as well as the Ohio State University in the USA. This was conducted by (Barraclough, Hay-Smith, Boucher, Tylka, and Horwath, 2019). For ease of reference, we will refer to this as Study One.

STUDY ONE

The object of this study was to teach more middle-aged women about intuitive eating and taking note of teaching techniques—what worked and what didn't, barriers to success and other obstacles faced in trying to embrace intuitive eating as a new way of life. Findings concluded that women found it extremely difficult to accept that there were no longer any restrictions on the types of foods they were allowed to eat.

This study also discovered the "social and psychological barriers" were the most challenging obstacles to get past.

Part of the educational process was allowing these women to move beyond the standard "good food, bad food" scenario and onto eating whatever they wanted, as and when they wanted, eating when they were hungry and learning to stop when they were satisfied. This proved to be a significant challenge to most within the test group.

The study determined there were definite improvements in feelings of health and wellbeing overall on both a physical and psychological level.

It proved problematic in actually teaching the test subjects what intuitive eating was all about and ensuring they understood it to make full use of it as a new lifestyle. Gaps in training were identified. In a number of studies conducted by nutritional psychologists, it was found that those who had participated in the "Mind, Body, Food" training found transitioning to eating by listening to their bodies far easier than following habitual eating patterns. Those exposed to these interventions (88%), found it to be useful (77%) and easy to use (68%) and said they would recommend it to others (84%)." (David, n.d.)

The test group consisted of only 11 women aged between 41 to 51, of different races, ethnicities, social and economic backgrounds. The results of the above study include the following, which have been revised and condensed for brevity:

INTUITIVE EATING VS DIETING

When dieting (on any form of diet) each of the women described their feelings as being guilt-driven or deprived. They also noted there were consistent feelings of being on a rollercoaster whenever they were dieting conventionally. In contrast, when using the intuitive eating method, they felt as though it was a much healthier approach to food.

"You can have what you want when you want. You just have to pay attention to when it doesn't feel good anymore and stop." *(Participant 11).*

Additional comments from participants included being able to quieten that voice that screams inside your head, telling you that what you're eating is 'bad for you.'

Others became more accepting of who they were resulting in weight loss almost immediately. Rather than berating themselves, they became more compassionate and self-accepting.

"The most moving part for me was that meditation about accepting your body. I cried. It's a COMPLETELY different way of thinking about your body than the one our culture seeks. Just appreciating the health of your body. I'm a really fit, active

person and I love being active. I really forget to value that." (Participant 5).

Some allowed themselves to now begin eating anything, while others stuck to their rigid 'good food/bad food' mantra.

"If I have a good breakfast and lunch, I could have something naughty for tea and not have to hate myself for it. I've learned not to feel guilty when I do have something that I know is naughty because I've given myself permission to enjoy it." (Participant 4)

Some women embraced this new diet free lifestyle, while others still questioned why they had not lost any weight. They admitted to having more energy and vitality.

HEALTHY FOODS AND INTUITION

This area was not as clean-cut as above as many of the participants battled with where to draw the line on what foods were healthy for them, or simply eating anything until their bodies let them know they were full.

For one of the participants, she discovered that by listening to her body, she was able to feed her body the specific foods it craved at the time—often being the right foods.

DNA OR UPBRINGING?

Many participants felt that they should have been taught the right way to eat by their parents, rather than having to relearn it all over again now. Others felt that we have been conditioned by the world we are currently living in, one that is fast-paced and offers freshly baked, delivered, fast food virtually everywhere you look. While this may be convenient, it does nothing for an intuitive eater.

Because the world has changed so drastically, many of us that fall into this midlife point need to be re-trained to eat correctly, rather than settling for a burger or pizza that can be delivered right to your door. For some this is comfort food when facing an emotional crisis. This is especially when it's necessary to remain strong and focused on getting your mind and your body working together. Taking a stand against the voices in your head and going in search of food that's actually going to make you feel better both inside and out.

Learn how to become more aware of your own feelings towards certain foods. Begin to savor and enjoy them, rather than quickly gulping them down so you can move onto something else you need to tick off your checklist for the day.

CHILDHOOD FOOD PHOBIAS

If you are like me, you grew up in a home where dinner was a family affair at the dining room table. There were no cell phones to interfere with daily conversation and nobody got to leave the table until everyone was finished eating everything! If there was something you didn't like, you had to suck it up and eat it because the alternative was way worse than the taste of spring beans or Brussel sprouts! If you were fortunate enough to have a family dog that you could secretly pass the food onto in a completely innocent way, you may have left the table unscathed. The alternative was spending hours chasing food around your plate with a fork in the hope that someone was going to insist on leaving the table.

The fear of retribution for not eating *everything*, and I mean EVERYTHING on your plate at every meal often imprinted on us and has carried itself with us way into adulthood. To this day there may still be certain foods you cannot stomach, and they actually result in a negative emotional connection with that specific food. Being able to detach yourself from this will leave you feeling in control and empowered once more, rather than guilty for feeling the way you do.

REMAINING FOCUSED

Part of the final section of this case study was encouraging and allowing each participant to consistently reassess where they were on their journey and remaining focused on intuitive eating. It was getting them to discover what was deep within them that they could utilize as a means of winning the psychological war against food.

Other members of the control group discovered that it was easier for them to work together with the rest of the members in the group. This was done by being able to connect and network with one another, reaching out when they felt they were about to face a low, or 'fall off the wagon'. They found this camaraderie helpful to provide and receive support from their team—knowing that they weren't the only ones out there who occasionally felt they were losing the war.

Others discovered different techniques to help them overcome their negative body thought patterns and behaviors, also by sharing. This, in turn, helped their mental and psychological well-being and gave many of these women a new lease on life. For many, taking part in this group of test subjects gave them a platform to be of service to one another, discovering that they had a lot to offer others, rather than wanting to be on the receiving end all the time.

FOOD AS A LOVE LANGUAGE

Many of these participants began to realize that there was way more to food than just consuming 3 to 6 meals a day (or whatever your specific needs indicate). They found that approaching the way they viewed food changed their entire outlook towards socializing with others. It increased their willingness to share meals with friends and other family members, without feeling guilty about over-indulging. Better food choices were normally made right at the beginning, preventing unwanted, uncomfortable feelings. By relying on intuitive eating, this experience was once again something to look forward to, rather than dreading holiday get-togethers and the accompanying guilt caused by overeating. Intuitive eating also gave them the power to decide what foods to eat at these festivities—instead of being pressured to dish up something from every plate passed before their eyes. It returned the power of choice as to what to eat and in what quantity.

STUDY TWO

This study consisted of a much larger group of 2,287 younger adults with the average age being approximately 25.3 years old. The main focus of this study was body mass index (BMI) and potential eating disorders that could be associated as a result of intuitive eating (Denny, Loth, Eisenberg, and Neumark-Sztainer, 2013).

Males indicated that they could pick up from their bodies when they needed to eat, as well as how much they needed to eat. The females in this group of studies reported finding it more difficult to know when to eat and when to stop.

In most cases within this study, BMI was not affected at all and those who were able to get their intuitive eating patterns down showed no signs of eating disorders. On the other hand, those who could not tell when to start or stop eating (i.e. they had no idea how to listen to that inner voice within them), were more susceptible to binge eating or chronic dieting.

The same study indicated that long-term dieting is also not a solution. Instead, an alternate healthier way of eating and/or lifestyle is what is needed.

This study also found that being forced to eat everything that's been put on your plate as a child could have much longer-lasting negative effects into adulthood. And so the cycle continues—we demand the same from our children because it's how we have been raised.

Some of the results of this study concluded that we were able to regulate our food intake from a young age (infant), and we continued to do this as a toddler until it was forced out of us. We need to be able to get back to this point again where we can hear that voice that lets us know when we're actually satisfied. We need to listen to it and apply it to our daily lives, not just short term, but as a way of life.

Our bodies know exactly what we need, when we need it, and how to burn what we have stored. Unfortunately, it can't do this if we keep getting in our own way. There has to be a point where we begin to trust our instincts and intuition once more. Allowing that voice to come through and paying attention to what it is saying to us.

WHY ARE WE EATING?

These doctors and professors suggest three reasons why we eat. Think about each of these carefully as you put the next morsel of food into your mouth:

1. Am I eating because I am really hungry?
2. Am I eating because that food smells really good and it's making my mouth water?
3. Am I eating because I'm feeling sad, mad, glad, guilty, or alone?

By being able to identify which of these three categories you fall within, you may begin to decipher what is driving your eating mentally and emotionally right now. You should actually only eat because of the first factor – that of hunger!

HOW DO YOU FEEL?

In his blog (2012), Brian Johnson quotes renowned dietician Marc David as suggesting in his books: "The Slow Down Diet" (2005), and "Nourishing Wisdom" (1994) that we take a closer look at factors influencing us while we eat. Eating out of fear could make us either more fearful or guilty. An example of this would be switching to healthy food to prevent yourself from becoming ill. He also suggests adding another question to the above: how does eating this food make me feel?

Are there psychological factors you may be going through at the moment that may be influencing your current relationship with food? How do you feel about your life in general?

David divides all diets that you could possibly think of into four distinct areas. This could also influence intuitive eating by eating from the place where you're listening to what your inner voice is telling you. These four areas are:

- **Experimental**—don't get stuck on one eating style or set of menus permanently. Every now and again, experiment with exciting new styles of cooking and eating. You may just discover that there are other foods out there that you prefer to eat. These new tastes may excite you and unless you show signs of allergies, you may be able to add entirely new menus to your routines. It can also break down monotonous meals that are actually boring you and potentially robbing you of joy that you should be feeling over mealtimes.

- **Maintenance**—you may be very happy with your current body weight and shape; your BMI may be exactly where you'd like it to be. This is where a maintenance diet is handy. You don't want to do anything extreme by changing too much because this could result in picking up unnecessary weight. At this stage, it's time to batten down the hatches and simply see your diet through. No matter how mundane or boring.
- **Optimizing**—you would be considering an optimizing diet if you were getting ready for a marathon or some other major sporting event where your health and energy levels need to be at their peak. This would result in replacing certain food groups with others. You may need to be loading carbs that you can burn during activity.
- **Therapeutic**—as the name suggests, this style of eating would be especially helpful while recovering from some form of illness or trying to boost your immune system. An example of this would be preparing for a potential flu season by increasing your intake of vitamin C through oranges and guavas. These could be turned into a delicious early morning smoothie to start your day just right.

2

IDENTIFYING THE PROBLEM

"Throw out the diet books and magazine articles that offer you the false hope of losing weight quickly, easily, and permanently. Get angry at the lies that have led you to feel as if you were a failure every time a new diet stopped working and you gained back all of the weight. If you allow even one small hope to linger that a new and better diet might be lurking around the corner, it will prevent you from being free to rediscover Intuitive Eating."

— *EVELYN TRIBOLE*

Just as any good therapist would begin a treatment session, the initial challenge when it comes to intuitive eating is being able to identify food problems you are currently experiencing. It means stepping out of that comfortable space and looking at all the ways you and your body could benefit from learning as much as you can about intuitive eating. What better way to do this than to turn to the experts that got this ball rolling?

Being able to clearly identify where you are with your relationship towards diets and food is the only way to begin to move forward. This is not going to happen overnight—instead, it's a process. It's going to require that you step outside of yourself (or definitely back from your current situation) and analyze the way that you behave and your attitude to food.

This can be much harder than it looks, but there are some ways for you to get started.

DON'T JUDGE YOURSELF

Without being too harsh on yourself or judging yourself in any way, take into consideration your eating habits, behaviors and attitudes. We are normally extremely hard on ourselves when it comes to self-judgment and feeling the need to be perfect in every way. In many instances, this need is what drives our body image.

Ignore the voices of anybody around you with something negative to say concerning your physical appearance. These individuals will always exist. One of the keys to intuitive eating is self-acceptance and learning that you're okay just as you are, rather than having to conform to fit in with what the rest of the world brands as acceptable.

It's what's inside you that counts way more than physical appearance. In intuitive eating, once you've been able to master this challenging phase, your mood, self-image, self-esteem, and self-awareness will each receive the massive boost they need for you to begin to accept yourself as you are. Only then can you begin to become more relaxed and this is when losing weight can begin.

Ask yourself whether you are feeling physically hungry, or whether you need to eat because you are suffering from some form of psychological problem. There are distinct differences between the way these two forms of hunger present themselves.

PHYSICAL HUNGER

Your body is generating signals that it needs food and nutrition at any specific time. Physical hunger is something that occurs biologically within yourself. The symptoms of physical hunger come with physical cues that are given by the body. Some of these cues include your stomach physically growling or rumbling to coincide with feeling empty. You may feel faint and lightheaded or dizzy. For some, headaches accompany this state of hunger. They may even become irritable or show signs of nausea. When physical hunger occurs, the body needs something to ensure it can actually keep going.

If you've been able to confirm that your hunger is physical hunger, then try and rank it on the fullness scale we discussed in Chapter 1. Remember that you're trying to feed your body when it reaches the stage of hunger, rather than starving. Your body will be satisfied with whatever food it's given. This sets it apart from binge eating. When you've eaten something, stop when you are comfortably full, rather than once you've overindulged. Learning to listen to that internal voice can be really difficult at first because you need to drown out everything else you're being bombarded with by the world. Everywhere you look around you, new diets, fads, gimmicks and miracles are being promised as the next best thing to give you the perfect figure, size or weight!

This is the point where you actually need to call "Bullsh*t" on each of these empty promises, because that's exactly what they are. They are there to make money off of you and keep you trapped in a perpetual state of dieting.

KEEP TRACK

It's time to start tracking exactly what you're putting into your body and when. Keep an accurate journal of your eating habits. Begin this food journal without judging yourself. You're aiming to gain a better understanding of the types of foods you're consuming and when. You're also looking for trends in behavior and/or attitude, while not trying to reach any conclusions as to what you're eating or why.

Record as much information in your food journal as possible. This could include things like whether you drank water or a soda; was the soda sugar-free, or an energy drink? Were there specific times of the day where you felt your body hitting a particular "low"?

Working with the sliding scale we've already discussed, record the point that you were at when you started eating, and when you stopped. The ideal is to start when you're feeling hungry and stopping when feeling comfortably full (around 6 or 7), rather than stuffed.

Include how you were feeling on the 1-10 scale. How did you feel afterward?

Being able to review this journal after a few weeks could show patterns or trends beginning to emerge regarding specific foods or food groups that you enjoy eating. You will be able to clearly see whether your liquid intake consisted of fruit juices, smoothies, or energy drinks, rather than choosing water instead (which the body needs daily to be able to function).

IS YOUR HUNGER EMOTIONAL?

Are you eating because you're emotionally drawn to food right now? Do you see food as a means of escaping your current situation? When this hunger appears, what types of foods seem to make you feel better about yourself?

Once you've given into the temptation of "comfort food", how are you feeling about yourself? Do your choices bring on thoughts and feelings of guilt and shame? Additional side effects of emotional eating usually result in low self-esteem because comfort food is seldom healthy food. How many times have you suffered from emotional hunger and thought to yourself, "Ah, I'm off to get myself a healthy salad"? More often than not, it's everything that we should be avoiding, or at least not going all out and overindulging in. Those chocolates aren't really going to make you feel better about yourself. Nor will that tub of ice-cream. Emotional overeating results in you feeling worse about yourself in the long run because you've packed on additional pounds that were unnecessary.

Emotional overeating is a short-term fix to other deep-rooted problems, but the overarching results of unwanted weight gain could leave you feeling even more depressed.

CAUSES OF EMOTIONAL OVEREATING

There are many reasons responsible for emotional overeating. Emotions that could lead to overeating include, but aren't limited to stress, anxiety, depression, losing a loved one, divorce, changing jobs, loneliness, post-traumatic stress syndrome (PTSD), to name just a few. Along with this list, any number of things could trigger a change in the way you feel emotionally. Let's just say that being faced with emotional hunger is like a fuse in a powder keg of dynamite just waiting to be set alight.

Some of them are out of our control, however, our response doesn't need to be to reach for the junk food. Stress is a major cause as indicated, in a letter published by Harvard Health Publishing (2018).

According to research conducted in a survey by the American Psychological Association, approximately 25% of Americans rate their stress levels to be above 8 on a 10-point scale.

The risk factor of the body remaining in a constant state of stress is that the "fight or flight" mode kicks in. Unfortunately, when we're in this emotional state, digestion shuts down, making it more and more difficult for any food consumed to be digested correctly. This "fight or flight" response produces high levels of insulin. This prevents food from being broken down correctly, resulting in weight gain and obesity.

When someone is in a permanent state of stress, additional chemicals are released through the adrenal glands. This is known as cortisol and acts as an appetite stimulant. You can begin to see the problem: you have an increased appetite constantly, but the body's digestive system is in lockdown mode. If you are constantly under extreme stress, all these sugary, sweet "comfort foods" should rather be avoided, or replaced with something that's a healthier option. With all this additional cortisol, feeding the body is necessary, but with the digestive tract affected, processing these foods correctly is a challenge.

COMFORT FOODS

These are all those foods that we reach for or 'crave' when we are having a hard time mentally, physically, or emotionally. It's that packet of chips with the rich dip on the side, it's giving in to the chocolate donuts that call out to you as you do your best to walk past the bakery while en route to another store. It's that tub of chocolate chip ice-cream that has your name on it and calls out to you at the same time late at night. Giving in to any of these foods that have no nutritional value is akin to behaving like a small child with a security blanket. As long as it's there, everything in the world is okay.

Being able to turn to these foods, or anything like them whenever we feel the urge is not healthy for us: this leads directly to binge eating.

BINGE EATING (OVERINDULGENCE)

According to the Oxford Dictionary (n.d.), binge eating is considered to be *"the consumption of large quantities of food in a short period of time, typically as part of an eating disorder."*

It's estimated that this condition affects nearly 2% of the population (Mandl, 2019). Those suffering from binge eating disorder normally present with at least three of these symptoms:

- Eating alone because they feel embarrassed or ashamed
- Eating excessive amounts without feeling hungry
- Eating rapidly
- Eating until uncomfortable
- Suffering from feelings of guilt and/or disgust towards themselves

Because of the above symptoms, people who engage in binge eating find it particularly difficult to come to terms with their body image. This continues to spiral downwards with more guilt and unhappiness every time they go through another binge eating phase. Most find it difficult to break this cycle without some form of therapy or counseling. In many instances, both psychotherapy and counseling are required over an extended period of time before the patient can overcome binge eating.

Research is still thin when it comes to actual causes of binge eating disorders, although much of the research is readily available (PubMed, n.d.). Some causes may relate to both gender and general health. Statistics in the United States indicate at least 3.6% of women will suffer from a binge eating disorder at some stage, while only 2.0% of men will experience the same thing. It's also thought that it could be a characteristic that's passed on genetically.

Other major factors include how we think and feel about our weight and/or body. Whether it's size, shape, or form, if we're not entirely happy with what we look like or feel like, we stand a higher chance of experiencing binge eating at some stage during our lives.

What's interesting about this report is that dieting can be a major trigger for binge eating and if you've suffered from it in the past, there's a strong possibility of relapsing.

RISKS ASSOCIATED WITH BINGE EATING

If all of the information above isn't enough to convince you that binge eating is bad for you, there are a number of potential health problems that could arise from binge eating disorders if left unattended. These include, but aren't limited to:

- Asthma
- Cancer
- Chronic Pain Conditions
- Diabetes
- Fertility Challenges, including polycystic ovary syndrome (PCOS)
- Heart disease
- Insomnia
- Irritable Bowel Syndrome (IBS)
- Obesity
- Stroke
- Type 2 Diabetes

Often those suffering from binge eating disorders aren't even aware that they have this problem. Many of them raid the refrigerator in the middle of the night or make themselves a snack at strange hours when they're supposed to be sleeping. As to whether they are aware of their actions or not, it still constitutes binge eating and is unhealthy for both physical and mental well-being.

EATING BAD FOODS

When it comes to dieting there are always certain foods or food groups that are completely off-limits according to most of the diets out there. Once again, evidence-based findings are identified by what these "bad foods" might include, as well as the reasons why.

While there are many foods that can help you to lose unwanted extra weight, there are others that make losing weight virtually impossible. The eleven foods are identified by Palsodottir as the following:

Beer/other Alcohol—Further studies report that the energy content in 1 gram of alcohol is 29kJ or 7.1 kcal. While in some instances drinking wine in moderation may be healthy for you and assist in losing weight, excessive drinking of other alcoholic beverages could lead to weight gain according to the International Life Sciences Institute, (2013).

There was a direct link to weight gain where heavy consumption of spirits occurred, although this study revealed that further investigation was necessary to identify which specific types of alcohol presented the highest risk. When it came down to it, overindulgence and heavy drinking habits seemed to be the major factor determining potential weight gain and alcohol intake.

Chocolate Bars—one of the biggest contributors to weight gain, with an average-sized bar containing around 200-300 calories. Most also contain added sugars, oils, and fats. This is usually something that most people add to their shopping carts as they reach the cashier because these are strategically placed there to tempt you to add these items as a last-minute purchase. They are strategically merchandised right where you can be tempted to add them as a final purchase. These chocolate bars are often the number one "go-to" when it comes to comfort food.

If you happen to crave something sweet in the chocolate category, it's best to look for dark chocolate with a high cocoa percentage. As a caveat when it comes to chocolate, always read the labels. You may be shocked by the amount of sugar you're consuming that has no nutritional value whatsoever. All that it's doing is adding to your waistline and leading you straight down the path towards obesity.

Fizzy Drinks—most fizzy drinks and sodas have an extremely high sugar content that isn't processed by the body as food. As a result, no matter how many sugary, fizzy drinks or sodas you consume during the day, your body doesn't feel full at all. Drinking these drinks in large amounts on a daily basis can be hazardous to your health and general well-being. Soft drinks, or any drinks for that matter, are not registered by the brain as food. Although they are loaded with calories, your brain is not processing that you're ingesting any food. It's not registering when you're feeling satisfied, or full. The only way to get around this and being able to win the war against weight is by giving them up completely.

Because your body is made of between 60% and 65% of water, some of which is lost during the day and discarded as waste, perspiration and excreted as urine through the kidneys. Some of it is also lost due to digestion. This water needs to be replaced for the body to remain in optimum condition. Because of this, drinking water is essential for the survival of the body. Water is actually the only liquid that is recognized by the body as a liquid.

Foods with Added Sugar—many products labeled as being "low-fat" are potentially far worse for you because they contain much higher levels of sugar to camouflage the bland taste. Once foods have been processed to be "low-fat" or "fat-free," they lose much of the natural flavor that would be found in fresh produce. When in doubt, it's always a good idea to check out the labels to see actual nutritional values, rather than grabbing products off of the shelves that appear to be "good for you." Examples of these could include many types of breakfast cereal, granola, yogurts, cottage cheese, etc.

Fruit Juices—even the consumption of fruit juices in excess can be a risky habit to get into. While you may believe that those fruit juices that are labeled as 100% pure fruit juice are good for you, realistically, all that they contain is 100% fruit sugar, with none of the pulp (the good part) of the fruit. If none of the pulp is contained in the juice, there's really no point in consuming it.

Some of the best ways to ensure you get the nutrition you need from fruit juices is to go out and buy your fresh fruit from the local store or market and then to process it into a juice yourself. This can be done using a blender which makes certain that all the goodness is left in the juice. It makes for a delicious morning meal replacement, or even a late-night snack, rather than reaching for one of the junk food instead.

High-Calorie Energy Drinks (Caffeine)—hot or cold,

these are a big "no-no." These are readily available in the form of energy drinks and you can virtually find them anywhere. What may seem like a quick "pick me up" when you're needing to concentrate on getting through something or meeting a deadline. These drinks are loaded with caffeine, which is not only addictive but also extremely bad for you. Regarding these energy drinks, it's been reported that "in itself, caffeine is a stimulant, which, if taken on an empty stomach, can make you feel anxious and jittery. Because it's a stimulant it can increase both blood pressure and heart rate, negatively affecting you" (Brown, n.d.).

Energy drinks contain the highest levels of caffeine and are the most dangerous to your health and well-being. If you insist on drinking coffee, try and cut back to one cup a day and drink it black. Signs and symptoms that you may be addicted to your daily fix of caffeine may be suffering from headaches or experiencing irritability when deprived of caffeine. If you get to this point, it may be worth setting an appointment to meet with a health practitioner or dietician for assistance and advice to break your dependency or addiction to caffeine.

Ice Cream—another unhealthy item on the list of foods to avoid. This time because it is high in sugar and calories. The biggest problem with ice cream is that it is comfort food that is easy to consume in vast amounts in one sitting, rather than enjoying in moderation with long intervals in between. Consider limiting the amount of ice cream you dish up for yourself and limit the number of times you can enjoy it during the week or month. As you get into the habit of smaller portions, spread further apart, your body will thank you for it and you won't feel bloated all the time, or consumed by cravings that need to be satisfied.

Pastries, Cookies, and Cakes—because the main ingredients in these are refined flour and sugar, these should be cut back on substantially. It's convenient to stop off for a pie and fries at a local diner at lunchtime, rather than substituting this with a meal that may be healthier for you. Considering all the added sugar that can be found in cakes and cookies, most of the frosting alone is pure sugar, making it difficult for your body to process this amount of sweet food. Once again, a healthier option when craving something sweet is to choose dark chocolate with a high percentage cocoa ratio. This will satisfy your craving and is a much healthier option than conventional chocolate.

Pizza—due to the availability of this as fast food, it's extremely easy to opt for a pizza rather than physically cooking a healthy meal. Pizza is another food that has a base made out of highly refined flour and this combined with all the processed toppings, make it a ticking time bomb! If you really want to treat yourself to pizza, consider making your own at home and choose fresh, healthy toppings – that way you will know what you are eating, rather than accepting what is being handed to you by the pizza joint, where you have no control over where the ingredients have come from, how old they are.

Another problem with pizza is that we overindulge, forcing ourselves to eat the entire pizza in one sitting. If you feel the need to do this, consider scaling back and ordering one size smaller than you normally would. Your body will thank you for making this decision as you won't feel as bloated or disgusted once you've finished the last slice.

Potato Chips and French Fries—the best way to eat potatoes is by boiling them rather than roasting them or deep-frying them. One study on PubMed was conducted between 1986 and 2006 with 120,877 women and men in the USA. Each was assessed over four-year intervals and baselines were adjusted to factor in changes in lifestyle etc.

The results indicated that over each four-year interval an average of 3.35lb was gained mainly as a direct result of eating potato chips. This research concluded its findings to include things like lifestyle changes being linked with the increase in weight gain. This study also showed that most of those with excessive weight gain also consumed alcohol, smoked and did not have a strict exercise regimen.

White Bread—this falls within the scope of refined foods and also contains a lot more sugar than the body needs.

A study conducted in Spain evaluated some 9,267 university graduates for a period of 5-years taking their dietary habits into consideration. After a baseline had been established over 136 different items of food in a questionnaire, changes were monitored and reported annually. Weight changes were recorded specifically surrounding weight changes linked to portions of white bread consumption. By the end of this study, it was found that those who had consumed more than two portions of white bread daily were at direct risk of being either overweight or obese (BMC Public Health, 2014).

TAKING ON NEW DIETS THAT HURT YOU MORE THAN HELP YOU

For anyone who has weight issues or a problem with accepting their body image, dieting is always in the back of your mind and whether you realize it or not, your subconscious is constantly on the hunt for the next magic "fat-melting solution" or "magic pill/potion" that will get rid of the unwanted weight, rolls and flab overnight.

Unfortunately, there are more con-artists out there who are only too happy to oblige and provide you with something that has apparently been tested somewhere in some far off place and promises that it's 100% natural, with no side effects, yet will get rid of all of your unwanted extra pounds overnight. I use the word "unfortunately" at the beginning of this paragraph because thanks to us, these unscrupulous individuals manage to remain in business and even prosper until someone actually does the research into their products and debunks them as another fad or myth!

What you need to understand about diets that are available out there is that there are more than what I could possibly list in the remainder of this book. However, what makes diets and dieting challenging for all of us is that each of us is unique and has unique needs. It's the fact that your DNA is different from my DNA that separates our ability to react the same way to a diet. In addition to this, we may possess other underlying conditions that hamper dieting rather than help it.

Some of these conditions include problems with our thyroid. This could either result in overactivity or underactivity of the thyroid gland. Not only is the thyroid responsible for regulating the metabolism throughout the body but when it's overactive, the following could be experienced:

- Anxiety
- Arthritis
- Diabetes
- Insomnia
- Premature greyness
- Restlessness
- Vitiligo—loss of skin pigmentation

By not understanding everything that is going on in your body, it's simply too risky to get involved with any diet that's not recommended by a medical practitioner. What's even better is to consult with a certified dietician who can assist you with meal planning according to your specific requirements.

WHY WORK WITH A DIETICIAN?

There are a number of reasons to work with a qualified, certified, and registered dietician. The most obvious reason is that they are experienced in this field. Often more so than your normal General Practitioner, or other doctors or therapists. A dietician can work directly with you, refer to your medical history and any recent operations that you may have had. They can take into consideration any chronic medication that you might be on, especially those drugs that have side effects that lead to weight gain. Once you consult with a dietician, you will be surprised by learning how many medicines have weight gain as a possible side effect. If you've been on these treatments for any length of time, it can become more and more difficult to get the body's metabolism back to the point where it's able to lose the weight you have gained.

Just hearing this from a qualified professional can provide us with hope and the knowledge that we can do something about it. A dietician is not going to put you on a "diet" per se: what they normally do is get you eating correctly by focusing on a balanced diet. In many instances, this is exactly what the body needs for its metabolism to begin to function correctly once more.

3

HUNGER IS THE ENEMY

"Instead of indulging in 'comfort food,' indulge in comfort meditation, comfort journaling, comfort walking, comfort talking, comfort manicures, comfort reading, comfort yoga, comfort hugging."

— *KAREN SAMALSOHN*

Probably one of the most challenging aspects to face when on a diet is the hunger pangs that continue to strike. These occur because your body is simply not receiving the right amounts or sources of nutrition necessary for it to function correctly. This is what dieting does. It often starves the body of being able to process the correct nutrients necessary for the body to function properly.

An important factor here is being able to recognize when your body is hungry, feeding it the correct type of foods in the right amounts and regularly enough to sustain and promote good health. Too often when people are on a diet, they allow their bodies to move into a state of starvation before feeding it. This leads to consuming large amounts of food quickly, without actually tasting it and appreciating it for what it is. What this course of action is doing is removing the joy and happiness from the meal and merely replacing this with 'stuffing the food down as quickly as possible.'

HUNGER PANGS AND ROUTINE

The danger of eating in this manner is that hunger is often present at times of the day that fall outside of our 'routine.' This is something that needs to be accepted and honored, rather than ignored because it's the incorrect time to fuel your body.

This is especially true of patients suffering from diabetes—it's better to regulate food intake to 6 smaller meals per day than sticking with 3 meals a day, as this may lead to times where the body is ravenous, to the point that sugar levels drop, and the incorrect foods are consumed in an attempt to give the body what it needs to be able to function correctly.

ARE THERE REALLY CAN'T TOUCH FOODS?

The single most important lesson in this section is that food in itself is not good or bad. You are also not good or bad because of what you do or don't eat. If you are eating intuitively, you could even plan ahead for a treat once or twice a week. This will do a lot to ease feelings of guilt, which then spiral down to feelings of anxiety, depression and stress due to poor food choices.

Eat until you are no longer hungry, and no more.

Listen to the signals of comfortable fullness when you feel you have had enough. As you're eating, check-in with yourself to see how the food tastes and how hungry or full you are feeling. This involves taking your time while you are eating, paying close attention to what the food actually tastes like. To do this we may have to learn to put our knife and fork down during our meal, chew food more thoroughly and drink water as we go.

Most of us focus on getting through a fully loaded plate of food as quickly as possible, without actually spending much time focusing on the texture or taste of the food. We don't spend much time enjoying what we eat or considering what each individual item on our plate tastes like and how it makes us feel! Does it bring us joy? Do we ensure that we remain 'present and in the moment' as we eat? Or are we eating just for the sake of eating? This is where intuitive eating and mindful eating virtually cross paths. It helps us to bring ourselves into the present moment as we enjoy each meal, rather than seeing how quickly we can get through whatever's in front of us so we can move onto the next activity scheduled in our day.

RESPOND TO HUNGER VERSUS ROUTINE

Learn to respond to early signs of hunger that you may be feeling by feeding your body when you are feeling hungry rather than at a specific time. For many individuals, a routine of 3 large meals a day can lead to overeating and gaining weight. If we were raised in a home where you weren't allowed to leave the table unless your plate was completely empty, this could result in weight gain due to overeating.

Learning to feed your hunger as you become aware of it, is much healthier for you to give your body the nutrition that it needs when it needs it. By letting yourself get to the point where you are excessively hungry, you are much more likely to overeat.

DROWN OUT IDEAS OF GOOD AND/OR BAD FOODS

This is another philosophy that's instilled in us from the time that we are adolescents moving into adulthood—the fact that certain foods are good and other foods are bad. In addition to this, you are not defined as either a good or bad person based on the food that you are putting into your body.

Too often young children and teenagers are taught by teachers at schools, magazines and often even parents or peers that 'you are what you eat' and by eating certain foods you are heading down a particular path towards obesity and self-destruction. For really young children, this can cause the early onset of body complexes. Many find it really difficult to get over these beliefs when planted subconsciously from a young age.

While many of these individuals are well-meaning, it's ultimately not their choice to make and they are also not aware of your specific body's needs. When you begin to eat intuitively there's no such thing as one food that's better for you than another. Consider how a diabetic needs to maintain their insulin levels throughout the day in order to function normally. By being forced to stick with a strict diet, this can actually do more harm than good. The foods that have been identified by the diet as being 'healthy' for a normal individual, may prove to be unacceptable for those suffering from underlying conditions. Too many times we deprive ourselves of those things that are exactly what the body needs because we are following a 'diet' to the letter. We don't recognize a craving as something that the body specifically needs. There's a difference between satisfying a craving and overindulgence. One would be wise to be able to identify where the fine line between the two begin and end.

CHALLENGE THOUGHTS THAT TELL YOU OTHERWISE

Whenever you hear a nagging voice in your head that this food should be avoided, or that you need to delay eating at this time because it's not the 'appropriate hour' for you to be eating—challenge these thoughts. Banish them from your mind completely and remind yourself that it's these thoughts that have led you to where you are right now. Unhappy with life and especially unhappy with your body image.

Once you can get these feelings under control and you can allow yourself the freedom of eating when you are hungry, even if the foods are something you would have considered bad before, you will truly be back in control.

While you are challenging your thoughts on whether or not you should eat and when, ask yourself whether your hunger is physically motivated (genuine hunger), or emotionally motivated (there's something deeper going on). If you find that it's emotionally motivated, try and figure out what the emotion is that's behind it and how it's connected to the food(s) you are craving?

Are you eating out of loneliness? Do you feel guilty about something? Are you punishing yourself for something? Observe how you feel about your binge eating session once it's over? Chances are that you are going to be even more unhappy and unforgiving towards your actions and your choices of food!

THE NEGATIVE EFFECT CAUSED BY CULTURAL BIAS

Society has a huge role to play in how we feel about ourselves and the negative body image syndrome that many of us suffer from. As mentioned before, the tabloids and society at large are responsible for the cultural biases that recommend that we should look and behave in a certain way. Unfortunately for society, we are all different and cannot fit into the 'cookie-cutter' mold that they would like us to conform to.

This can be extremely pressurizing for many individuals who feel the need to fall within the parameters of this model. Especially when they are big-boned, heavy-set, have a specific body type and also other pre-existing conditions preventing them from being able to conform to the 'ideal'. It is mainly women who fall into this category, and the failure to be able to conform to the ideal body image as portrayed and/or projected by society, the greater the pressure to do whatever it takes to get there. Namely, diets, pills, fads and exercise programs that don't work for most people.

Many of these diets have not been researched sufficiently, and there is not sufficient medical and/or scientific evidence to back up the claims. Far too many individuals spend thousands of dollars annually on trying to achieve the perfect body type or body image they so anxiously desire. When these diets take too long or result in addiction to the "miracle drugs" themselves, the long-term results become even more harmful to those following these diets. Intuitive eating, on the other hand, allows you to decide for yourself what your body wants and what you'd prefer eating, rather than having a diet dictate what you can and can't eat.

SOCIAL MEDIA PRESSURE

Whether we care to admit it or not, we've all got friends on our various social media accounts who seem to have the perfect body and the perfect lifestyle. While they may not intentionally want to rub your nose in it, each time you scroll on your news feed, you can't help feeling totally pressurized by all the ways you don't seem to measure up to them. Each image on their Instagram account makes them look like they've just stepped out of the cover of *Vogue* magazine.

Others are constantly physically active, participating in marathons, cycling events, or other forms of extreme sports. When it comes to comparing ourselves to them, we are maybe not doing ourselves justice. It's easy to see a 'perfect lifestyle' when you're not getting the full picture.

The danger of comparing yourself to others in your social circle is that it could force you further down the guilt and shame spiral. If all that you can focus on is how much you fall short, or fail to live up to the expectations of others, you could easily get stuck in your own head. When you're in this space, you become limited in your ability to recognize those things around you that can bring you joy. Your vision becomes myopic and centered on your short-comings. You become aware of your bulging waistline, the fact that you can no longer fit into your favorite jeans, the fact that you are quickly out of breath simply walking around in a large shopping mall.

This comparison trap is exactly that. It's going to paralyze you where you are and prevent you from physically doing something about it. In truth, we can't all be a size 2. For some of us, there are underlying health issues that limit movement and prevent us from signing up with a gym, getting involved with high impact exercises, participating in marathons, or getting involved in team sports. We need to accept that as much as we are all unique, we also have potential limitations that could be difficult to overcome. As long as you are making an attempt to do something, accept that comparing yourself to others is unrealistic. It can add to feelings of insecurity and poor body image: all those things that you're trying to work through and move past.

As long as you allow your mind to control your body image, especially through comparisons, you will find it more difficult to accept yourself for who you are and make peace with all the positive things your body can do.

4

IT'S ALL IN YOUR HEAD!

"Accept your genetic blueprint. Just as a person with a shoe size of eight would not expect realistically to squeeze into a size six, it is equally futile (and uncomfortable) to have similar expectations about body size. Respect your body, so you can feel better about who you are. It's hard to reject the diet mentality if you are unrealistic and overly critical of your body shape."

— *EVELYN TRIBOLE*

How you feel about your body image, whether you're pleased with yourself or whether you can't stand looking at your stomach, thighs, or arms—it all starts in your head. Your conditioning is all psychological and once you can identify where and when all of this started, you have a starting point to begin to repair your thoughts and emotions.

MENTAL HEALTH

Mental health is an extremely important factor when it comes to accepting your body image. Without positive mental health surrounding your body, you will be drawn to diets, overindulgence, or even binge eating: it will influence your normal eating habits and possibly even lay the foundations for your children's body image down the line. If you can accept that your body image is all in your own head, you can begin to fix it.

Your negative body image may be as a result of someone teasing you about being a chubby child. While they may have been joking with you at the time, you may have taken their teasing to heart and allowed yourself to be negatively influenced by this name-calling. This may have made you feel negative towards yourself and your body, causing you to begin your dieting crusade in search of the perfect body so that you would never be called a 'chubby kid' ever again.

Learning to accept yourself for who you are is the first step in learning to fix those things about yourself that you don't like very much. Start off by making two lists: a list of those things that you like about yourself, and one of those things that you don't like about yourself. Once you have completed both lists, find someone who you trust, who knows you well, and ask them to be objective while going through each of your lists. You can also get them to add anything else to either list.

They can also cross an item off of your lists and either replace it with something else or give you a reason why they've made the change. You may be pleasantly surprised by how different these lists can actually look. One of the main reasons for this is because we are permanently in our own skin and are too close and judgmental of ourselves. We can't see all the good things about ourselves. Instead, we spend endless amounts of time and energy criticizing ourselves daily for things we either can't change or issues that aren't there to begin with because they're actually all in our heads.

Not accepting ourselves for who we are can leave us filled with low self-esteem which in turn leads to increased levels of stress and anxiety. It's only by accepting who you are, as you are, that you can begin the process of healing and becoming whole again. Once you are able to sort what's real from what's going on in your head, it becomes a little easier to start breaking down some of these mental barriers holding you prisoner in your own mind.

RESPECT YOUR BODY

We are quick to judge and pick up on our shortcomings with our bodies, especially our perceptions when it comes to what we believe is wrong with it—our arms are too short, our toes are ugly, our thighs are covered with cellulite, our butts and stomach are too big and out of proportion. While we are so busy focusing on all of these negative things, we cannot see the wood for the trees, so to speak.

You cannot see your strengths where you perceive weakness(es) to be, or opportunities where before you have only seen failure. Your body is capable of so much more than you are probably giving it credit for. You are probably excellent at so many things, but the harsh judgments you hand down to yourself because of small shortcomings put you at such a disadvantage when it comes to your mental health.

Try and find the beauty in parts of your body. In some instances, you may be so negative about your body image that this is a monumental challenge to overcome.

An example of this is a friend of mine who teaches health, fitness, yoga, spinning, aerobics and aqua-aerobics at a local gym. Since she was a teenager, she has always paid close attention to her health and has been the epitome of fitness. Even now, being super-fit, completing cycle tours and long-distance marathons, she is extremely aware of her own body. Here's someone who has no reason for any negative self-image issues towards her body. She's correctly proportioned, her body mass index (BMI) is ideal, she works out every single day and is toned and tanned in all the right places—yet she hates her body!

She's acutely aware of everything about it, often comments that she wishes she were different and finds faults where there aren't any to be found. I can only begin to imagine how many other individuals are out there who have similar beliefs or feelings towards their perfectly sculpted bodies. This is one of those examples of where a negative body image has been formed and fueled by the mind.

In reality, people would do anything to have her problem of being stuck in a perfect body, yet these individuals see themselves completely differently, maybe as a result of something that happened to them as a child, or an adolescent. Trauma may have occurred that's preventing them from moving forward past this point, and all they can do to control it is to engage in self-loathing and hatred towards their body image and shape.

The right thing to actually be doing if you are in this situation is to start celebrating your body for the many things it is capable of, and recognize just how beautiful parts of your body could be just as they are.

HONOR FEELINGS

Learn to honor your emotions for what they are as and when they arise. Don't give in to using food as a means of coping with any emotions whatsoever. Trust yourself and your body to find other ways of dealing with feelings and emotions—that don't relate to food. There are so many other things that you can be doing rather than binge eating. You need to try and find alternate ways to cope and alternative things to do in the time available that's going to keep you as far away from food as possible. Some ideas are, but not limited to:

- Journaling
- Meeting up with, or calling a friend
- Going for a brisk walk
- Meditating
- Doing crafts
- Trying to learn new skills

The important message to get across when you're feeling this way is to replace the hunger that you're feeling with an activity instead. It's learning to recognize that your hunger is coming from an emotional place. If your hunger is emotion-based, you need to be able to identify the emotion and try and trace it back to where it comes from. Does it have a specific trigger or cycle that it follows? Is it something that occurs daily? Are there specific times of the day when you feel more emotional hunger than others? Is there something else that is causing this emotional hunger to be triggered at this specific time of the day?

TAKE TIME OUT

Something that's important when it comes to switching to intuitive eating is to learn to slow down when eating. This involves not just eating for the sake of eating and getting finished as quickly as possible, but rather learning to savor the food that you have in front of you. It's relearning how to enjoy what you eat, rather than gluttony.

Choose foods that you enjoy and are going to bring you pleasure. Take the time to actually sit down at a dining table to eat your meals, rather than eating your meals on the run. Learn to eat more slowly, savoring the taste and texture of the food on your plate. Take short breaks during your meal, allowing the food to digest properly. This will give your body the time that it needs to let your brain know when you are satisfied. This can't be achieved when you sit with a plate that's piled high and you tackle it like it's the last meal you're ever going to have.

Learning how to eat this way can help your body communicate to your brain once it is satisfied and has had enough. This is the point where you need to physically stop eating. Don't carry on eating because of childhood traditions where you were forced to clean your plate. You will find that eating becomes a genuine pleasure. Discovering foods that you like or don't like will become easier to do because, maybe for the first time since you were a child, you will probably be able to come to terms with each variation of food on your plate.

You will bring the power of eating back into your own hands once more, rather than feeling the need to be force-fed whatever is on your plate. You will rediscover the joy of eating, as well as not having to eat more than your body requires. Your body will also begin to learn that if it should begin to feel hungry, it will be fed with something that it enjoys. This is truly the art of intuitive eating. Less food will be able to satisfy your hunger, and you may find that there are certain new foods that are more appealing to your palate.

5

EXERCISE - THE WAY TO LOOK AND FEEL BETTER

"Even when all is known, the care of a man is not yet complete, because eating alone will not keep a man well; he must also take exercise. For food and exercise, while possessing opposite qualities, yet work together to produce health."

— *HIPPOCRATES*

Instead of embarking on high-intensity body workouts or signing up at the nearest gym to go all out, think about ways to get your body moving initially that will help you feel better about yourself. Contrary to popular beliefs, there's a lot more to exercising than just burning calories that you've consumed.

BENEFITS OF EXERCISE

Finding the right exercise to meet your needs is as important as deciding what foods work for you. The benefits of exercising are as follows, but not limited to:

BALANCING YOUR WEIGHT

Combined with intuitive eating, exercising plays a vital role in helping you control your weight. It also prevents obesity. The best way to maintain your weight is to ensure that the calories you eat and drink equal the energy you expend during the day.

If you are trying to lose weight, the calories consumed as a result of the physical exercise and your daily movement (this includes everything, even cooking and cleaning) need to be higher than the number of calories consumed during the day. Having said this, there's more that needs to be factored in when it comes to wanting to lose weight. Metabolism and any health morbidity should be taken into account. Be kind to yourself when looking to shed some extra pounds. After all, intuitive eating is about loving yourself and accepting your body image for what it is: weight loss is not the goal.

IMPROVING YOUR MENTAL HEALTH

The opposite of exercise is immobility and can normally best be described as lying on a couch or doing nothing particularly productive with your body. This leads to some serious health problems including obesity and heart disease; more importantly it has a negative effect on your mental health as a whole.

Too often, we fail to connect the dots between a lack of physical exercise and a positive mental attitude or our mental health in general. During exercise, the body releases chemicals that improve your mood and make you feel more relaxed. These chemicals are known as endorphins and can help you deal with feelings of stress. They can also reduce the risk of feeling depressed. This is one of the reasons why so many diets insist on a combination of exercise together with the diet.

Exercise also prevents you from focusing on negative things happening around you as you are having to pay attention to physically doing something else instead. According to Gingell (2018):

- Exercise can treat chronic mental health issues.
- Exercise reduces depression.
- Exercise in some cases can be as good as pharmaceutical interventions (this is a huge benefit for those suffering from chronic illness who have been on medication that actually adds to the patient's weight problem, often resulting in drug-induced obesity).
- Exercise can be used to help with anxiety, dementia, depression and even mild cases of schizophrenia.

KEEPING THOUGHTS SHARP

Exercise can also stimulate and release additional chemicals and proteins that improve the functioning of the brain. It can stimulate learning, keep thought processes sharp as well as improve rational decision-making as you get older. Being in better control of your brain and thought processes can help you when it comes to intuitive eating. You will definitely be able to make wiser food choices.

Over 39 different studies concluded that memory

skills and the ability to think clearly were drastically improved for those who exercised regularly (BBC, 2017).

Australian researchers (in the same study) commented that it was worthwhile beginning to exercise at any age: so, if you think that you're too old to begin doing something about your health right now, think again. It was recommended that those who could not take on extremely challenging forms of exercise for whatever reason, try Tai Chi as an alternative.

Findings of this study especially focused on some of the major benefits that could be achieved through regular, consistent exercise, no matter how old the individual or how simple the exercise, the following results were detected:

- Growth hormones, blood supply including oxygen were pumped to the brain.
- Cognitive abilities were improved--some of these included, learning, thinking, reasoning, reading, and reasoning.
- As long as physical exercise was part of the individual's routine, no matter what type of exercise it was, there were signs of improvement.

The ideal recommendation from this study was that regular aerobic exercise was engaged in, to increase the blood flow and oxygen to where it was needed in the body. However, if this wasn't possible, some exercise was better than no exercise whatsoever. Other recommendations included trying to fit at least 150-minutes of aerobic exercise into each week wherever possible.

IMPROVING SLEEP PATTERNS

Regular exercise can help you to fall asleep faster and remain in a relaxed state of sleep for longer. This in turn will help you make better food decisions. Instead of reaching for that caffeine-loaded energy drink or espresso first thing in the morning, you should be waking feeling refreshed and ready to take on a new day without having to rely on anything else to do so.

Dr. Charlene Gamaldo, the medical director of John Hopkins Center for Sleep at Howard County General Hospital, stated following a recent study that "We have solid evidence that exercise does ... help you fall asleep more quickly and improves sleep quality" (John Hopkins Center for Sleep, n.d.).

She further mentions that the time you choose to exercise could impact this ability to sleep properly and that you need to take these into account. For some, exercising too late in the day may leave you too energized, making sleep more difficult.

She recommends (as do the previous studies) that moderate aerobic exercise will likely result in what's termed slow-wave sleep, or deep sleep. This is actually the type of sleep our bodies require to be able to recharge and rejuvenate, getting us ready to face whatever challenges the following day may hold.

She also confirms that exercise can stabilize our moods, allowing the brain to relax to the point where the correct form of sleep is possible.

According to her research, there are two factors which could affect sleep depending on when we exercise during the day:

1. **Aerobic exercises** - endorphins are released which could result in you needing to remain awake. To move past this point, she recommends that you should exercise at least 2 hours before retiring to bed. She clearly states that "the brain needs time to unwind."
2. **Core Temperature** - whenever we exercise, the body's core temperature is raised (similar to when we take a hot shower). The endorphins released send signals to the brain that it's time to wake up. It usually takes anywhere between half an hour to an hour and a half for the body to return to normal temperatures.

Try and figure out what your inner clock tells you regarding exercise, so you are aware of how late you can exercise before trying to get some sleep. This is something that only you will be able to recognize and decide for yourself. Nobody can prescribe exactly what times you should be working out. In the immortal words of Shakespeare's Polonius in Hamlet - "To thine own self be true."

One of the most important things to consider when trying to improve your sleep patterns is that you exercise long enough for your sleep to be positively influenced. Dr. Gamaldo recommends about 30 minutes of aerobic exercise for you to begin to feel the difference in your sleep patterns. She also states that the benefits of exercise will begin to be felt almost immediately.

Find some form of exercise that you enjoy doing; that way you will be motivated to continue with it on a daily basis. Begin slowly at first, especially if you are overweight or obese. You don't want to overdo it on the first day so that you feel as though you never want to exercise again.

When it comes to improved sleep, the returns are almost immediate. You will also begin to feel better about yourself for doing something to make a difference to your own health.

BEGIN WHERE YOU ARE

So, you may be wondering to yourself how you get up off the couch (which is usually your favorite spot to vegetate), and start exercising? The answer is simple—start off slowly. You don't want to go all out immediately because you will burn out quickly or injure yourself, doing your body more harm than good. Remember that you need to be able to respect your body and honor it where it is now.

If you are currently overweight or obese, understand that it took a long time for you to get there, so don't expect a miracle to happen overnight. The excess weight that you're carrying around with you isn't magically going to disappear the moment you begin exercising. Part of being kind to yourself and your body is learning that this is a process and one that's going to take time. Patience is a habit you are going to need to develop and master as part of your 'no-diet' journey into intuitive eating.

Even thinking about where to begin on this road to recovery can be absolutely daunting. These feelings can be fear-based out of self-loathing towards body image. You may not want to appear in public (at a gym) and face up to others whose bodies seem perfectly toned and balanced.

Other reasons for putting off any exercise routine could be out of fear that it's going to be painful to try and push through because you already know that your body is in such bad shape that you don't have the strength to do most of the exercises.

So where do you start if you fall into this category? The American Heart Association (AHA) recommends at least 150-minutes of moderate exercise every week (Timmons, 2016).

This may seem an impossible task, even breaking it down to 30-minutes per day for five days... But, what if this was broken down even further into bite-size chunks that could be managed? Say, 10- or 15-minutes at a time? This is beginning to sound less daunting already. Do what you feel you can manage realistically, without feeling as though you have to climb a mountain. If you manage to get short bursts of exercise in, these all add up in the long run. What's just as important as reaching the 150-minutes per week, is being able to see it through.

Start where you are. Look for ways that you can begin to exercise slowly and build up the strength and stamina necessary to get you going and into a routine. Even if you start and end each day with a brisk walk around your neighborhood. It's definitely a start and before long you will realize that this routine's no longer challenging enough for you. This is when it's time to step it up a notch.

Here are some exercises as recommended by the AHA that you could try and ease into:

1. **Stationary Bike Riding** - These bikes normally have a back-rest, making them ideal for those

who are overweight or obese. Because most overweight individuals battle with their core muscle strength being able to cycle on this type of bike can be the ideal starting point.

2. **Walking** - This is something that's low impact and can be done anywhere. You don't need to pay for it and you don't need any equipment, so even if you're away on business, going for a brisk walk is doable. Begin slowly and as you become fitter, you can increase your pace, distance and duration of your walk.

3. **Water Aerobics** - Very low impact on the body because your body is supported by the water. This has numerous benefits to those who may not be physically able to engage in long walks or cycling. Find a pool that offers water aerobics classes. You may be pleasantly surprised by how refreshing and enjoyable this type of exercise can be.

For someone just starting out, a combination of all three of the above exercises is recommended as they target different muscle groups.

EXERCISE ROUTINELY

As mentioned above, the AHA recommends 150-hours of physical exercise per week in order for you to lose weight or receive physical benefits from an exercise program. Starting is the hardest thing to do. Decide what you most want from your life. Making a decision to begin a simple exercise routine can work wonders for your self-esteem and will yield positive results and long-term improvements to your health and your life.

You are already aware that you're overweight or obese, or you wouldn't suffer from low self-esteem or a poor body image. You're not happy about the way that you look and the only way to make changes is by physically doing something about it. Realizing that taking the first steps towards exercising on a regular basis is one of the few things that are going to help you feel better about yourself is the first step.

You don't need to sign up to that Pilates class or join a gym (unless you want to…). The truth is much simpler: as discussed earlier, the key to being successful is to begin and begin where you are. Do things that are easy to incorporate into your life and your routine. If you have small children, take them for a walk with you in their stroller. You can walk around your neighborhood or walk to a local park. The pace that you begin walking may be slow at first and you may begin to feel your muscles tiring initially. This is exactly when you shouldn't stop because you are beginning to burn those calories.

Some other ways to incorporate physical exercise into your daily routine could be by taking the stairs rather than an elevator whenever the opportunity arises. This doesn't only need to apply to your work environment. Going to a meeting with a client on the 3rd floor? Take the stairs. After a while, you'll begin to feel like you can take on more and more flights at a time without tiring as quickly. Your muscles are starting to be strengthened, so is your stamina and your resolve to keep going.

Some other ways of introducing exercise into your normal, daily routine is by:

- Walk to a co-worker's office rather than sending an email.
- Wash your car on your day off.
- Park your car further away from the shopping mall so you have to walk more.
- Involve your friends and family—explain to them what you're trying to achieve and let them either join you or act as a cheerleader to your exercising cause.
- Get involved in classes that require exercise: try YouTube videos for Zumba or other classes, and follow these routines in the comfort of your own home.
- Take your dogs for a walk/run every day.
- Sign up for physical activity groups—volleyball, water polo, dance, hiking, kickboxing, figure 8 dance classes.

If you're just starting out in your quest to become physically fit, it may be worthwhile to try out a couple of different classes to see which resonates with you, before signing up and committing time and money.

Groups are a great way to go because the participants often act as cheerleaders to keep each other motivated.

TRACK YOUR PROGRESS

Keep a journal that can track your progress. This could include the physical activity you were engaged in, the amount of time you spent doing it, and possibly the way that it made you feel at the end. An example of this would be:

[Date][Physical activity engaged in][How long or how far][I feel...]

Nobody is suggesting that you make a novel out of this, rather keep a simple diary to monitor what you are doing. After a short while you should begin to notice that during the same period of time, you are able to achieve more. This is an indication that your body is beginning to get stronger and your stamina is improving at the same time.

An example of this would be if you were to begin walking. Initially you may only be able to walk for 10 minutes in a day without feeling uncomfortable or tired. After a month of regular walking, you may notice that you've been able to increase the amount of time that you're walking to 20 minutes and you've more than doubled the pace and distance.

You could use apps that you could download onto your phone that can help you calculate how many steps you walked for the day. Begin by setting smaller goals for yourself and increase these incrementally over time. As you reach each of your goals, celebrate each achievement. Once you've done so, set a new target so that you keep yourself motivated towards pushing yourself further constantly. Goals achieved need to be rewarded - try not to attach this reward to food though! Find some treat that you really want and reward yourself as you reach each of your fitness/weight goals. Replace what used to be a food-based reward with something else. An example of this could be booking a massage, buying a new item of clothing, treating yourself to a movie at the cinema.

These are the small victories that you should be aiming for. Some other tools that you could add to your arsenal against your negative body image are things like a tape measure, a scale, and even a mirror. Your clothes may give you another indication that you're beginning to shed some weight.

In your fitness journal, record how you are beginning to feel about changes you're experiencing, especially towards your body image.

PUT THE FUN BACK INTO EXERCISE

You are likely to get bored easily by repetitive exercises over a long period of time. You can overcome this by trying to bring the fun factor back into exercising. Apart from listening to music or watching TV while you work out, mix up your activities. Set up an exercise schedule that has some variety and try making changes to the schedule so that you aren't doing the same exercises each day.

Consider exercises that can be done year-round, taking the weather into consideration. If it's raining, find exercises that can be done indoors. The main point of getting into an exercise routine is being able to stick with it so it has a positive impact on your health and your weight. This is vital for a positive body image.

The main aim of exercising is to get the body moving, the blood flowing and to help you feel better about yourself. If the added benefit to this is weight loss, then this is a bonus. You are trying to ensure that your physical and mental health needs are taken into consideration.

Here are a number of other ideas that can easily be incorporated into your routine to spice things up a bit:

- **Dance like no-one is watching**. Being self-aware, especially when it comes to having a negative body image can be one of the toughest battles you will ever have to face when exercising. At some point, you need to just stop caring about whatever the rest of the world thinks and realize that you are doing this for you. Show up for yourself and work through the gamut of emotions that will come as you begin to become more physically fit. Don't listen to what anybody else has to say. Their opinions are not important: your health is!
- **Don't procrastinate.** It's easy to hit the snooze button in the morning and roll over going back to sleep rather than going for a walk, run, or engaging in your chosen exercise routine. This is where you need to be strong mentally and make a decision that no matter what happens you will stick with it. Decide that you aren't going to place your health on the back-burner any longer - instead, you are going to regain control over your life.
- **Find your reason.** Rather than exercising because you hate the way you look, use self-esteem, self-awareness and self-care as reasons to motivate you onwards and upwards. If you are battling with low self-esteem, do it for a loved one. This could potentially be for your spouse or your children. Set a goal that includes them as part of your reason for wanting to be more physically fit and healthy.
- **Try weights on for size**. A popular myth in

health and exercise circles is that if you are overweight you need to get cardio going first, before moving onto weight training. This is not true. You can begin with weights in the comfort of your own home. Another benefit of choosing to add weight training to your routine is that it works much quicker than cardio on its own. Training with weights will allow you to quickly notice that you are becoming physically stronger. As this happens, you will become more motivated to continue working with weights. Weights can also be adjusted according to how far you're ready to push yourself. You can add or subtract weights until you feel comfortable.

- **Sign up for a walk-a-thon or a race.** Look for those that have short distances that you know you'd be able to handle. Ask a friend to join you or involve your partner and your family. They are ideal motivators. Mark the date down on the calendar and place this somewhere prominent where you'll see it every day (like the fridge). You can often find charity events of this kind. Most of these are advertised on social media such as Facebook. All you need to do is commit to attend and put the work in to prepare to participate.

6

HOW DO I ACTUALLY EAT INTUITIVELY?

"Having a healthy relationship with food means you are not morally superior or inferior based on your eating choices."

— *EVELYN TRIBOLE*

HOW TO EAT INTUITIVELY

According to Rumsey (2017), there are five specific tips that she shares to improve the relationship we have with food. It all begins with getting rid of the misconception that certain foods are better than others, and that depending on what you eat you should feel guilty about it. Her five tips are to:

- **Forget about diets (all of them)** – all diets do is make you feel guilty about yourself and even worse about your body image. This is the antithesis of what you're trying to achieve. You want to begin to feel better about yourself. If you wanted to feel bad, you could go back and join all of these diet groups where you need to weigh yourself every couple of days, count how many calories you're eating within a day, etc. If you've made friends with these people via Facebook or LinkedIn and are watching videos on YouTube or listening to podcasts as to what you should be doing and how you should be doing it, I have two simple words for you —STOP IT!

You can replace these with those that promote anti-diet living instead. Some of these are listed below with the links in the reference section:

- Immaeatthat blog
- Rachael Hartley Nutrition blog
- The Foodie Dietitian blog
- The Real Life RD blog
- Food Psych Podcast
- Love Food Podcast
- Nutrition Matters Podcast
- The Nurtured Mama Podcast

- **Understand and use the Hunger/Fullness scale** – we've covered this in previous chapters, but this scale can be quite challenging to come to terms with initially. The biggest challenges occur in being able to tell when you are actually feeling hungry (when the correct time it is to eat), and when you've had enough to eat (when you are satisfied but not overstuffed).

Getting this balance right takes time to master. It's about learning to eat slower, to actually enjoy the food(s) that you are eating when you are eating them. It's also about taking regular breaks during your meal to analyze how 'full' you are feeling at the time. This is so that you get to recognize when you are feeling comfortable and satisfied, rather than uncomfortable because you've overeaten. This is the most challenging part of intuitive eating.

Discovering exactly how you feel in terms of fullness or satisfaction and then honoring these feelings by putting your knife and fork (or spoon) down. It's moving past that old mentality of having to eat everything on your plate simply because it was placed there.

- **Eat exactly what you want to eat** – the reason why this pointer is so powerful is that it breaks the 'diet' mentality completely. It no longer restricts you with those foods that you can or can't eat. You can throw out the list of all the things that you have up to this point considered to be 'bad' for you. Suddenly the physical 'craving' of certain foods is removed because the barrier or ban on eating them has been lifted. Have you ever been on a diet where you weren't allowed 'ice-cream' and found yourself craving it multiple times a day? Eventually, at some stage you would cave and go on an all-out ice-cream eating binge, only to hate yourself for doing so the next day!

If you think about this psychologically—when there are no barriers to hold you back regarding those foods that you can or cannot eat, the pressure of having to fill the empty void of craving is gone. That ice-cream may be a small treat for one day of the week or once every two weeks. You aren't physically removing it from the equation and placing labels on foods—making some good and some bad!

PRACTICE MINDFUL EATING

Rumsey (2017) continues by suggesting that you practice 'mindful eating' – this is where you pay close attention to what you are eating, where you are eating (your surroundings), and what each mouthful of food physically tastes like. It's like starting a taste bud revolution and discovering the taste of foods as if you were eating them for the very first time.

To eat mindfully you need to be able to slow your eating patterns down considerably. Physically taking the time to chew each mouthful of food properly. Allowing your taste buds to work their magic. What does the texture of the food do to your mouth? How does the food make you feel?

Mindful eating involves physically sitting down at a table and ONLY eating. It's not multitasking by eating in front of the TV, or computer. It's also not grabbing your meals on the run while you rush out of the door, late for that business meeting or appointment and you have your briefcase in one hand together with the car keys and a croissant in the other that you can gulp down in the car on the way. It's also definitely not stopping through a fast-food drive-through on the way home because you're exhausted from your day and you just know that cooking is the last thing you want to do once you get home.

When you master mindful eating, you'll begin to notice when you're hungry, and also when your body is satisfied. You'll treat your body with more respect as you take your time with each meal, focusing on the food itself and the way that it's making you feel. This will replace current unhealthy habits that you have with food at the moment, with ones that are going to be more beneficial to you in the long run.

CHALLENGE THE FOOD POLICE

Her final tip is to challenge the 'food police' running around in your head! This is those voices that keep challenging you with what you can and can't eat. These voices have been around for a long time. For many of us, most of our lives (or at least since we were teenagers and began all these see-saw diets).

How can you recognize the food police? Easy—whenever you hear a nagging voice in your head telling you that you shouldn't have eaten this or done that! These are the voices that make you feel guilty and inferior. Sometimes they can bring self-loathing and guilt with them – telling you that you are fat and/or ugly and nobody will ever be able to love you!

We mentioned keeping a journal and a logbook for your exercise. Another journal may be a good idea to begin tracking these negative internal thoughts that you have about yourself. Whenever you recognize any of these thoughts entering your mind, write them down. You can then begin to pull them apart and physically analyze them. Where do they really come from? Are they real? What is the pay-off for this kind of thinking? Make this journal an active part of your day and go through it often. You may discover that certain patterns begin to emerge that are linked specifically to either a specific time of day or a particular food. Once you discover this, they become easier to face head-on and deal with one at a time.

ONLY YOU CAN DECIDE

Up to this point, you may have thought that you have no control over what you eat, how much you weigh and your self-image. This is simply NOT true! If anyone has the power to change anything about yourself, it's you and only you. You are the one who needs to decide and make the necessary adjustments to meet your own specific needs.

In intuitive eating, the main rules are to eat only when you're hungry and to stop when you're feeling satisfied (rather than stuffed). It's using your 'intuition' or 'common sense' to do so. While this sounds fairly easy to do on paper, in reality it's way more difficult because finding and listening to what your intuition is telling you to do is often drowned out by the voices of the world.

The glossy magazines, billboards, social media advertisements, television, movies and everything else out there want you to feel bad about not having the 'perfect look.' What is the 'perfect look' for you anyway? You know your body, you know your bone structure better than anyone, therefore it makes perfect sense that this whole 'perfect look' thing should be left in your own hands.

It's time to stop listening to what everyone else around you are saying and doing. It's time to begin ignoring what the world wants and figure out what's going to make you happy. Once you've managed to do this for yourself, you will begin to feel more in control of where your life is headed.

RECOGNIZE AND FEED YOUR HUNGER

Hunger plays a key role in intuitive eating. It's the time that you should be giving your body enough nutrients, energy, and food that it needs in order to survive and thrive. There are two different types of hunger though and you need to be able to tell them apart.

Physical hunger happens naturally throughout the day at regular intervals. Depending on your body type, your physical health and any other underlying conditions which you may be suffering from, this hunger may need to be fed anywhere between 3 to 6 times daily.

If your hunger is connected to your emotions, try and find another outlet or way of dealing with whatever's going on with you. Identify the emotional trigger and attempt to work through it. This type of hunger is easy to fuel with comfort food (which is almost always exactly what you should avoid). Emotional hunger is what leads to binge eating and it's this that packs on the pounds because emotionally you're more inclined to retreat, rather than taking any form of action. It's this hunger that causes you to retreat to your bedroom with that tub of pistachio ice-cream and a spoon—leaving you feeling totally guilty in the morning!

Find ways to overcome emotional issues by choosing to be physically active instead. Get out, breathe in some fresh air and go for a brisk walk: it's better than sitting around feeling sorry for yourself. Most of all, be kind to yourself. Accept that you are feeling something that needs to be worked through. Journaling can often help to work through these issues as well.

CHOOSE FOODS WISELY

With all of your food choices, try and include as many fresh fruits, vegetables, and other staple foods as possible into your diet. This is normally where we fall short. We fill ourselves with too many processed foods that have no real nutritional value and can't satisfy physical hunger. Aim to include as many fresh foods as possible in your daily menu. Consider foods that are seasonal, as nature has a way of providing us with all the nutrients we need when we need them. There's a reason why certain foods are seasonal. Citrus grows mainly in the cooler months. Being rich in vitamin C, these fruits can help strengthen immune systems and help prevent colds and flu.

This may require doing some research but try and find those fruits and vegetables that are seasonal. Nuts, legumes, tubers and even meats are required to be balanced in our diets. Find what works for you. As long as the body is receiving all the nutrients it needs to survive and thrive. Fresh is always better than processed or frozen wherever possible.

BENEFITS OF INTUITIVE EATING

According to Jennings (2019), some of the major research-based benefits of intuitive eating are:

Those following intuitive eating plans have more positive attitudes towards lower body mass index (BMI) and weight management versus weight loss. This was according to studies published in PubMed (n.d.)

Improved psychological health, self-esteem and quality of life. This occurred because they had a better self-image making them less susceptible to anxiety and depression. In addition to this, these women were inclined to maintain the distance once following an intuitive eating plan. This was completely opposite of a regular diet mentality according to a study conducted by Schaefer and Magnuson (2014).

This same study also showed that following this kind of program led to long-term behavioural changes when it came to eating.

A third study completed by Ricciadelli (2016) indicated that those women who managed to master the art of intuitive eating were far less likely to display other eating disorders.

While much research has already been done on intuitive eating to date, there is still much that needs to be done to support these findings and more.

7

MY 5 STEP PROCESS TO SUCCESS

"Your body needs to know consistently that it will have access to food—that dieting and deprivation have halted, once and for all. Otherwise, your biology will always be on call, ready to avert a self-imposed food deprivation."

— *EVELYN TRIBOLE AND ELYSE RESCH*

In their bestselling book, Tribole and Resch challenged every major belief that dieting up to this point in history had claimed to be. In this book, they focused instead on providing a solution for those individuals who had tried diets and failed hopelessly. They provided a 10-step plan to challenge old belief systems and introduce new methods of thinking.

In an attempt to simplify their process even further, I'd like to provide you with the following five steps to get you motivated towards making healthy changes in your life that can have a lasting impact. These steps are not merely a fad or a phase to be adopted for a few weeks, only to be abandoned at the first sign of failure. Instead, they are meant to keep you motivated in building genuine life-altering habits that will become a lifelong commitment towards permanent change.

STEP 1: HOUSTON, WE HAVE A PROBLEM

Identify that you have a problem with consistent dieting, a poor body image, low self-esteem, or addiction towards trying on every single new diet or fad that comes onto the market. As with anyone suffering from any form of addiction, the first step in the recovery process is admitting to the fact that you have a problem in the first place. Own it and accept it.

- Recognize what this addiction is doing to you.
- How is it affecting you, mentally, physically and emotionally?
- How is it affecting your relationships with others?
- How long have you been unhappy with your body image?
- Is this preventing you from living your best life?
- Identify every negative sub-problem that's accompanied the diets.
- How much money have you spent over the years? (This could be on anything from gym memberships to lotions, potions, diet pills, and equipment including trainers, sweats, etc.) This financial figure should be enough to send you reeling!

- How much time have you wasted preparing all these diet meals and concoctions?
- How much time have you wasted reading labels while shopping and then paid twice as much on items because they say 'low-fat' or 'sugar-free,' only to discover that they're actually loaded with more sugar than the normal product (artificial sweeteners)?

STEP 2: ACCOUNTABILITY

Accept accountability for your own life. For your thoughts, feelings, and emotions. Analyze and recognize where your thoughts, feelings, and emotions are coming from when referring to your body image. Where did it start? Is it real? How has it affected you over the years? The key to this step is doing a deep dive into your own head. You'll be surprised by just how much of your low self-esteem, poor body image, frustrations, and emotions have built up over many years. You can probably trace the roots back to that one instance where that person happened to pass the comment about you being a "chubby kid."

Finding the origin of your belief system can help you to figure out what you need to be doing to heal yourself. Or at least where you can begin to challenge these beliefs. When we are young, it is easy to accept whatever we are told, especially if we were raised in an environment where you were forced to eat a specific way. These formative years can potentially shape us into dysfunctional adults.

You may have become addicted to dieting during your

younger adolescent years—not quite sure how to deal with body changes during puberty. Step 2 is all about getting to the root of your dieting dilemma. Discovering where it started. Only once you can recognize the beginning, can you begin to unravel the chords that are keeping you so tightly bound to constantly being at war with your body image.

STEP 3: DITCH DIETS FOR GOOD

We've learned from Evelyn Tribole and Elyse Resch (1995) that diets don't work and that it's way more important to listen to what your body is telling you. The people who managed to get off of the dieting merry-go-round are much happier, healthier individuals. They no longer count calories or try to figure out how much extra time they need to spend working out at the gym because they enjoyed a small slice of cake at the office celebrating a colleague's birthday!

Intuitive eating is all about recovering from yo-yo dieting and learning to become more intuitive by listening to what our bodies tell us about ourselves. It's figuring out what foods we prefer. It's about learning to slow down and appreciate our food for what it is, nutrition and fuel that the body needs to survive and thrive.

STEP 4: EMBRACE INTUITIVE EATING

Intuitive eating is not intended for the body to specifically lose weight, although weight loss may come as a natural by-product of eating correctly. Instead, it's about creating a positive body image for yourself so that your self-esteem is enhanced, and you are treating your body on a holistic level.

Getting into the habit of intuitive eating could assist you to shed pounds because the body is no longer in 'starvation' or 'stuffed' modes, which is exactly what many of these diets do. They create environments of either 'feast or famine' and the body is never certain where it stands. This is what leads to fatty deposits building up in the body as it stores food as a spare supply because it's not sure when it will be fed again! This is one of the biggest challenges and experiences that the body physically undergoes during a diet.

In intuitive eating, there will always be food there when the body feels hungry, and it will be able to have enough food until it's satisfied. It no longer needs to store extra fatty deposits—this is what could potentially lead to natural weight loss with intuitive eating. Accept and understand that intuitive eating is NOT A DIET!

STEP 5: IN IT FOR THE LONG HAUL

Accept that you need to give intuitive eating a chance to work and that it's not going to make major changes to your body overnight. Yes, you will certainly feel the benefits of being able to eat when you are hungry. The challenge is learning to read the cues that are going to tell you when to stop eating. This is where you need to become patient and eat slower, savor each mouthful—chew your food slowly. Enjoy each mouthful as if it were the last.

Commit to seeing intuitive eating through for at least 90 days. Avoid being tempted to hop back onto the next new dieting craze, just because it's there. Practice the techniques that have been included in the previous chapters, as well as those that follow. Your goal is to learn to love yourself and make peace with the relationship that you have with food. Remember to stick with your notes and keep on journaling on how eating intuitively is making you feel about yourself. For example, you can use these questions as prompts for daily journaling.

- How are you feeling about your relationships with others as a result of intuitive eating?
- Are you feeling more comfortable in your own skin?
- Is it easier for you to accept your current body image?
- What else has this journey taught you?
- How can you ensure that this becomes part of your life moving forward?

8

STOP BLAMING YOURSELF

"The Dieter's Dilemma is triggered by the desire to be thin, which leads to dieting. That's when the dilemma unfolds. Dieting increases cravings and urges for food. The dieter gives in to the cravings, overeats, and eventually regains any lost weight. He is back to where he started, with the original weight —or higher. And once again the dieter has the desire to be thin ... and so another diet begins. The Dieter's Dilemma is perpetuated and gets worse with each turn of the cycle. The dieter is heavier and feels more out of control with eating."

— *EVELYN TRIBOLE*

WHY BODY IMAGE?

Up to this point, we have been focusing on many of the reasons why individuals find the need to follow the latest diet trend. It may surprise you to hear that the number one factor that leads to any form of dieting is how we perceive ourselves and our body image. This is what we see when we look in the mirror. Our reaction to this image may be realistic, or it can be flawed. It's this flawed image that leads us to dieting, even from a young age.

We have an image of what we 'should' or 'shouldn't' look like on the basis of what society is telling us, what our parents are telling us, what our peers are telling us or a variety of other reasons. This is not to say that any of these reasons are true and correct. Breaking free from the bonds of body imaging is the aim of this chapter. I hope that you will gain greater understanding and appreciation for your body as it is now and learn why dieting is not the answer to changing the way that we feel about our bodies.

THE BODY IMAGE CONCEPT IS FLAWED

Statistics reported by The National Eating Disorder Organization (n.d.) indicate that awareness and concern for body image can begin in girls often as young as 6-years old! Girls between six and 12 are already worried that they're too fat. This is according to the publication by Thomas F. Cash and Linda Smolak entitled "Body Image, Second Edition: A Handbook of Science, Practice, and Prevention." (2011). This leads to looking for solutions by beginning to diet from such a young age. Some children turn to extreme diets and destructive behaviors that can range from smoking to taking laxatives, eventually developing eating disorders. Some unfortunately even go as far as developing anorexia nervosa or bulimia as they search for acceptance from their peers. Even the children who don't go on to develop serious issues become addicted to the diet mentality from an early age and unless the cycle is broken, this will follow them throughout their entire lives.

The only way to break this cycle is by learning to accept and love your body exactly as it is. It's learning to be grateful for the things that your body is able to do. How it supports you and carries you throughout the day. How you are able to move in a certain way, unrestricted and unhampered. It's being able to express gratitude and celebrate what you have, that many other individuals possibly don't have.

THE PERFECT BODY IS A FANTASY

Who or what determines what the 'perfect body' looks like? Is it a particular proportion? Facial features? Body shape? BMI? Is this decided by society? Peers? Parents? Or is it all in the mind? Should this decision actually be left to anyone other than yourself? Surely the perfect body or ideal body image is when we can get to the point of being comfortable in our own skin. Rather than benchmarking ourselves against celebrities, online influencers, or those lean, mean, toned 'models' promising you instant results if you just buy that shake or follow that diet. This is why buying into the whole dieting mentality doesn't work.

There are only so many people who are born with the perfect genetic makeup and body metabolisms that can process the food that they eat at a rapid rate, ensuring that they always look slim or lean. For others, they really work hard to get there and maintain a strict lifestyle of exercise and balanced food intake. This is completely different from following a strict 'diet' regimen to get to where they want to be.

They aren't sacrificing foods to stay fit—they've balanced their food intake according to what they are burning off during any given day's exercise, whether this is at the gym, running, swimming, playing golf—you get the idea!

They are not restricting their meals in any way: they have just learned what works for them and so can you. They are not fanatical about how they look, they are more interested in how their bodies can function.

WHEN DOES IT BECOME A DIET?

Any style of eating that restricts you from certain food groups or limits your intake of calories, carbohydrates or requires that you cut out other foods such as proteins, fats, carbohydrates or even wheat, should be classified as a diet and must be avoided at all costs. The body needs everything to function at an optimal level and the natural reaction to being told that it cannot have a certain type of food is that the body will 'crave' that specific food even more.

Rather than following all of these diets, from Paleo to Weight Watches, all the way to Intermittent Fasting, it's better for your body image and yourself to get rid of any and all siren calls that promise miraculous results within a matter of days.

ACCEPT YOUR BODY AS IT IS NOW—CELEBRATE IT

Accept your body for what it is now and learn to practice self-love instead. This should replace self-loathing because this is what is leading you to your poor body image in the first place.

If you're a mother who's now carrying around some extra weight that you haven't quite lost since you've had your children—celebrate this! You've had the opportunity to bring new life into this world. Celebrate each milestone that your children reach and think of the joy that they bring into your life daily.

If you have the use of your arms and legs, celebrate this and be grateful for everything that you can do with your limbs. Be grateful that you're able to walk daily and keep your body moving. If you can still bend and stretch and are supported by your spine—be grateful and celebrate all the things you can do. If your spine allows you the simple pleasures of picking up your children, or doing daily chores, being able to reach for things in supermarkets or stores while shopping—consider those suffering from bone deterioration that are unable to do these things anymore. Think of those now limited as to how far they can walk each day, or possibly even being confined to a wheelchair.

If you can see and hear and smell—be grateful for these abilities to be able to appreciate the beauty of the world around you.

While each of the above may seem to be obvious things our bodies can do for us each day, how often do we actually take notice of them? Do we accept and appreciate what we are able to do, or are we so focused on our perceived faults and flaws that we can't see what we already have?

Take out your journal and begin to write down all the things that your body can do for you right now—you'll be surprised at how long the list is, and how liberated you will begin to feel afterward.

FORGET THE FANTASY

Fantasy, perfectly shaped and proportioned bodies that look like they have been sculpted by an artist are far and few between. Those that are have possibly taken years of professional coaching and training to get there. Believe me, no matter what anyone says in any diet book, article, feature, advertisement, or blog—there's no new fad or gimmick that hasn't been kicked around the block a few times for decades before (in some instances even for centuries).

Anyone promising you instant results is a fraud. There's no such thing. Learning to eat correctly and getting your body moving is the only way to go, and you are the only one who can get intuitive eating mastered effectively.

You know what your body is saying to you and you need to follow the signs and cues that it provides you with. Be prepared to move more than you've done in the past, if you want to begin to see results, but remember that intuitive eating is not a diet! The promise of weight loss isn't attached to this plan. It could potentially be a by-product of learning to listen to what your body is telling you.

Remember that people come in all shapes and sizes, life has always been that way. We cannot all resemble models on the cover of glossy magazines (nor should we want to). You need to recognize sales and marketing ploys, especially around the dieting industry to be exactly what they are - lies that we've been fed to believe we need their products to become acceptable.

LET GO OF THE NEGATIVES

Whatever negative body image thoughts you've been holding onto—it's time to let these go and let them go for good. This is actually way more difficult than it sounds, purely because most of us have been raised with a negative mentality towards our bodies from a young age.

Your current negative thoughts surrounding your body image need to be banished.

But how do you achieve this when your negative thoughts can become totally overpowering at times? Get that journal out once again and write down at least ten things you like about yourself. Whenever you find your mind wandering off to the 'dark side' of negative body image, go back over this list again. You may even want to print this list out and place it somewhere prominent where you can read it daily. This will help it become a mantra to your daily living.

Just as we've dealt with the 'food police' in a previous chapter, where you're able to ward them off rather than paying them any attention, you can follow the same trend whenever you are faced with negative voices that tell you that you have imperfections with your body. (As a sidebar

—even those who have the so-called 'perfect bodies' aren't 100% happy with how they look).

Another valuable tip is to see yourself as a full individual—that is, more than just what your body looks like from the outside! There are a lot of people out there who have bodies that look perfect, yet inside they are horrible people! Beauty is more than skin deep; it takes your character and personality into consideration as well. Never forget that!

Monitor social media messages—what are they really saying? And, more importantly, are they real? Call them out whenever they're fake. Remember that you determine what you choose to believe and listen to—not social media or any media for that matter.

Be kind to yourself. We live in a world that can be harsh, judgmental, and dominated by plastic people. Take the edge off of some of this hurtful mentality by being kind to yourself. So you've had a rough day at the office, instead of aiming directly for that tub of ice-cream and a spoon to comfort you—stop and buy yourself some flowers instead. They will last longer than the ice-cream and beautify your surroundings, making you feel better about yourself.

Be of service to others—it's true that when you are serving others you can often lose yourself. Your own imperfections and shortcomings can easily become swallowed up while doing something kind for someone out there who is in greater need than yourself. If you're not sure where to begin with this, look at contacting animal shelters, homes for abused women or children, or consider visiting the elderly in local hospitals or assisting community projects to clean your parks, schools, or beaches, all are worthwhile pursuits.

BANISH THE BLAME GAME

Whenever we begin to gravitate back to negative body image, we begin blaming ourselves, our parents, our loved ones, or anyone else who happens to be in the way for allowing ourselves to get like this—even that chocolate cake! Whether it's genetics or choices we choose to use as a hook, we have an innate desire to lay the blame somewhere, and most of the time it falls directly back on our own shoulders.

The moment this happens, a negative spiral begins moving us downwards and closer towards a host of eating disorders. This happens because someone needs to be held responsible for allowing us to become this way. We see our bodies differently. This image is often distorted and removed from reality and this distortion is often the cause of eating disorders.

EATING DISORDERS

Eating disorders can range from physically abstaining from food—starvation, to binge eating disorders and a whole host of others in between.

Anorexia Nervosa

One of the most dangerous of all eating disorders. It starts out with some type of 'harmless' diet and ends up with total starvation. Those with anorexia cannot see themselves as skin and bones. Instead, whenever they look in a mirror, the image that's projected back at them is someone who's morbidly obese! The sad truth about anorexia is that most cases take years to recover with extensive therapy and counseling, or they could result in life-long serious medical issues or even death.

Bulimia nervosa

Bulimia nervosa is another serious eating disorder that claims many lives each year. Although it is similar to Anorexia nervosa, the main difference is that those with bulimia actually eat and then physically make themselves ill by sticking their fingers down their throat. The danger with bulimia is that gastric juices pass back through the esophagus often causing permanent damage. These are serious eating disorders and if you have the tendency to engage in this self-destructive behavior to try and lose weight, please seek help in the form of professional counseling.

Bulimia can also cause death in extreme cases, due to cardiac arrest caused by the stress that the body is placed under while it lacks the necessary nutrients to function correctly.

Neither anorexia nor bulimia should be taken lightly. For many suffering from bulimia, laxatives can be used as a form of getting the body to physically purge whatever food has been consumed.

Opting for a self-administered colon cleanse in the hopes of losing weight can rob the body of the very nutrients, fats, carbohydrates, and minerals that it actually needs. When these laxatives are taken most of the time the body hasn't had time to digest what it needs in order to survive and thrive.

Binge Eating Disorder

We've covered this type of eating extensively in

previous chapters. Binge eating stems mainly from eating to fill an emotional need rather than a physical (hunger) need. This eating disorder leaves us with many emotional scars, especially guilt and self-loathing.

Diet Pills

While diet pills in themselves aren't an eating disorder, becoming addicted to them can be dangerous. Whether it's weight loss pills, supplements or laxatives, they can all have long-term detrimental effects if they are used excessively.

There are literally hundreds of pills on the market that promise immediate results. This is one of the main reasons why there are so many diets available in the marketplace at the moment. It's a multi-billion-dollar industry that's growing daily and one that doesn't show signs of slowing down or stopping anytime soon.

Fasting or Intermittent Fasting

Many believe that this is a way to regulate the metabolism or recharge it, getting it kicked back into high gear once more with the promise of rebalancing any hormones that are out of whack. The only way to achieve this is by honoring your body and what it is telling you. Not by starving it from time to time. All that this achieves is getting the body to store more fat because it knows that there will come a time when it's not going to be fed.

Restrictive Dieting

Any diet that says that you should avoid certain foods or food groups is potentially harmful. If you were to visit any registered dietician, they would provide you with a proper breakdown of exactly what your body needs to survive. You'd be amazed that there are still fats included in these balanced diets because the body needs them to operate effectively. If a diet prevents you from eating anything—toss it out!

Skipping Meals

This is as close to fasting or intermittent fasting as you can get. Once again, if the body is feeling deprived of food, it's going to move into the 'store for later' phase. This is where fatty deposits begin to occur throughout the body so that it knows it has enough 'fuel' for the next time it's deprived. Starting to get the picture on why cutting back or cutting out completely actually leads to weight gain?

Steroids and/or Supplements

Part of this multi-billion-dollar industry. Many of these have not been tested accurately or they are used incorrectly. Because many of these are new to the industry they cannot always be accurately backed up by clinical trials. Pumping the body full of these chemicals is not a good thing. Even meal replacements such as protein shakes are never as effective as actually eating foods that contain protein. These supplements always contain other additives and ingredients that could have harmful side effects on the body if they are used over an extended period of time.

Unbalanced Food Intake

This is where certain food groups are removed from your food intake completely. An example of this would be cutting out carbohydrates, or protein from your diet. By restricting these foods from what should be a normal balanced diet, the body responds differently and begins to store fat. Even the body's metabolism is affected.

The recommendation when it comes to all these types of diets is to ignore all of them and aim for returning to a healthier, balanced lifestyle where you aren't restricted with what you can or cannot eat. It's learning to embrace food all over again and rediscover those foods that bring you joy. It's taking time to enjoy the food you're eating, learning how to savor it. When you reach this stage you will begin to embrace your body image for what it is and rather than feeling guilty or self-loathing, you will begin to replace these feelings with love, joy, and self-appreciation.

DEALING WITH DEPRESSION

Feelings of depression usually appear along with guilt attached to our eating habits. If we've 'broken' a diet by eating something on the 'bad food' list feelings of remorse can take over. These can begin with guilt as mentioned above but can quickly escalate to feelings of depression. This could lead to bouts of anxiety, panic attacks, self-isolation, low self-esteem and even self-hatred.

Depression can lead to complete withdrawal from society. Feeling too ashamed about our inability to remain strong enough to stick to a 'diet.'

This is no way for anyone to live. It's allowing your negative relationship with food to take over your life. By the time you reach this stage, you need to accept that you've moved past the point where you are in control. The 'diet' is now controlling you and you need help to get out of what seems to be a bottomless abyss of self-loathing, blame, and doubt in your ability to beat these feelings.

For some, you may have a strong support group to lean on who can easily coax you back from the edge and help you turn your current thoughts around. For others, counseling may be necessary. If you find yourself at this point, decide to change your Dieting Dilemma! Either turn to your support group and ask for help or pick up the phone and reach out to a professional counselor. This could be anyone from a Registered Dietician, to a psychologist or psychiatrist. Consider contacting your general practitioner in the first instance if you're experiencing constant low moods and feelings of depression.

Don't wait until you reach the point of no return. Know that there's always hope and help available out there.

HOW POSITIVE BODY IMAGE CAN ACTUALLY HELP YOU

We all understand the concept of the difference between something that's positive versus something that's negative. The same is true of how we feel towards our body image. When we can step back and appreciate our body for everything that it is and does for us on a daily basis, we may experience a positive shift in what we currently believe.

Understand and accept that we are all unique and have a distinct set of characteristics and personality traits that we can offer the world.

We have each been born to be unique and different and this is something to be celebrated. Imagine how boring the world would be if we all looked exactly the same, had the same measurements, wore the same shoe size, had the same eye color, hair color, skin tone, you get the idea. Can anyone say bland and boring?

Being different from each other is actually what sets us apart. It's why certain people are naturally drawn towards being more athletic than others. It's what separates the nerds from the jocks. We can't all be actors or supermodels either. Imagine the world without individuals that have made unique contributions or still continue to do so: Mahatma Gandhi, Nelson Mandela, Florence Nightingale, Madame Curie, Steve Jobs, Sir Richard Branson, Bill Gates, Oprah Winfrey, and the list can go on and on.

What about the valuable contributions that are yet to come as a result of the rising generation(s)? Are these going to be stymied or placed on hold because people don't like the way they look? Or because they are going to crack under the pressure that society places on them to look a certain way, dress a certain way, act a certain way?

There is too much negative emphasis being placed on body image. It needs to be replaced by encouraging individualism and celebrating and embracing diversity, rather than demanding 'cookie -compliance to body image.

Breaking the mold is going to be up to you and it's going to be the values you instill in your children. They are watching and learning from you daily and these lessons will be perpetuated and repeated in their own homes with their own children someday.

If you are currently restricting your family's eating habits because you're following some diet, you run the risk of harming future generations when it comes to their perceived relationship with certain foods.

It's better to teach your children the basics of what defines a healthy lifestyle, as well as intuitive eating habits, and encourage them to make their own decisions (obviously only once they are old enough).

We need to get back to the point in time where we become as little children—eat when you are hungry and once you've had enough, leave the rest. The mentality that most of us were raised with was as a result of the Depression (where you weren't certain where your next meal was coming from—so you ate what was in front of you). Today, we live in an environment where our cupboards, refrigerators, and freezers are full. We no longer need to be concerned about scarcity.

9

SURROUND YOURSELF WITH THE RIGHT ENVIRONMENT

"Make food choices that honor your health and taste buds while making you feel good. Remember that you don't have to eat a perfect diet to be healthy. You will not suddenly get a nutrient deficiency, or gain weight from one snack, one meal, or one day of eating. It's what you eat consistently over time that matters. Progress, not perfection, is what counts."

— *EVELYN TRIBOLE*

INVOLVING FAMILY

Getting the entire family on board with intuitive eating could present a challenge depending on how old your children are. Naturally, the earlier you are able to start teaching them about eating intuitively, the better it will be for all. Should your children be very young though, it's important that you don't overwhelm them with too many food choices per meal.

At the same time if you dislike certain foods, avoid

passing this aversion onto your children, even subconsciously. Allow them to make their own decisions regarding food preferences (as long as these don't only consist of fast foods). The emphasis here is on intuitively eating while choosing mainly those foods that are going to provide you with a balanced diet that is nutritional.

EAT TOGETHER

Starting to eat intuitively as a family is a perfect time to revive the age-old tradition of sitting down and enjoying your meals at a dinner table together as a family. Before televisions were invented, families would gather around the dinner table and communicate with each other face to face on all sorts of topics. There were no cell phones that demanded our constant attention or tv programs that we had just to watch. Dinners used to be a time of bonding and learning new things. It was also a time to discuss things that happened during the day. Parents actually knew what was happening in their children's lives and mealtimes were a fun part of the day.

Meals were consumed a lot more slowly as a result of each member of the family communicating with each other. This is what we need to be aiming for once more. Actually sitting down for meals. You could even consider making the dining area a 'cell-free/technology-free' zone for the duration of the meal. Make the meal and communication the focal point of the time that you spend together. This will allow you to channel your intuitive eating by enjoying your mealtime experience. As you take regular breaks while talking, before simply placing another helping of food into your mouth, think about where you are on the hunger—satisfaction scale? If you are satisfied, don't force yourself to clear your plate. Listen to your body, and honor both your hunger and your fullness.

When introducing intuitive eating to your family, although you may be the one responsible for what's dished up on everyone's plate, it should be up to them as to how much they eat.

Remember the toddler theory of only eating to the point where they're no longer hungry... this is what you're aiming for and this should be where you're aiming to get your family to as well. Let them decide when they've had enough.

If you're concerned about food being wasted, dish up smaller portions with the view that everybody can always have more if they are still hungry. In theory, the bigger the plate, the bigger the portion size that's served. If you know that you're definitely eating way too much food at the moment, look at replacing your current plates with ones that are smaller, and try to dish up proportionately to the plate. Be careful not to overload the plate as this may once again make you feel as though you must finish everything that's been served.

ALLOW CHILDREN TO DECIDE ON WHEN THEY ARE SATISFIED

Don't force-feed your children or insist that they eat everything in front of them. Part of the growing into the intuitive eating experience is discovering what foods you actually enjoy. Your family mealtimes should be happy times—that way you will experience and associate joy rather than pressure with food and mealtimes.

Don't pressurize family members to eat if they aren't hungry. For example, say that one of your children returned home from football practice and ate a fair size lunch around 4 pm: he's certainly not going to be in the mood to face another full-size meal at dinnertime at 6:30 pm. However, it will be worthwhile for his dinner to be placed in the refrigerator or microwave for when he actually is feeling hungry.

Remember the golden rule of intuitive eating—eat when you are hungry!

STOCK UP WITH HEALTHY SNACKS

Other ideas include ensuring that there are ready to nibble on snacks in healthy portion sizes stored in your refrigerator for easy access. You can also add these to your children's lunch boxes for school.

Healthy snacks could include anything from fresh fruits such as apples, pears, bananas, oranges, to cheese wedges or blocks of cheese cut into cubes. Boiled eggs are also a great option for a healthy snack as they can provide protein: the same goes for small amounts of meat or chicken.

As an idea for a more filling snack, for example for children who are active in sports at school, consider preparing a chicken salad that has added croutons and hard-boiled eggs.

Encourage your children to eat as many fruits and vegetables in their raw format, as it's in their raw form that they contain the most nutrients, making them the most beneficial.

STOCKING CUPBOARDS

Adding to the above, choose to stock your pantry with good, wholesome foods as much as possible. Ensure you make it as easy and quick as possible for you and your family to be able to whip up a healthy and tasty meal. For example, you can stock up on tins of chicken and/or fish that can be added to a fresh pasta salad quite quickly for a boost of protein. try to reduce the number of unhealthy snacks you stock on as they could be used as 'comfort food' when you're having a bad day. This would include all the usual suspects like cookies, chocolate bars, potato crisps, candy, and anything with high sugar content. Limit the amount of ice-cream available at any time in your freezer, and possibly replace it with frozen yogurt, or frozen fruits that can be blended into yummy and nutritional smoothies.

I'm not advocating that you don't have some treats to enjoy as a family: remember that the secret to intuitive eating is to have everything in moderation. Once you are used to feeding yourself with what you want, when you want, you will find that you experience fewer cravings for sweets and fast foods.

CHOOSE HEALTH OVER FAST FOOD

As a result of the fast-paced lifestyle most of us live, we've come to rely too heavily on the 'convenience' of fast food to replace a structured, well-balanced meal plan. This is where things begin to go sideways. It's easier for us to call for a pizza delivery or Chinese take-out, or stopping by Burger King on the way home from work, rather than taking the time to shop for food and prepare a proper home-cooked meal.

If you do a little research on the nutritional values of the most popular fast-food options, just one click away, you will find that most are actually extremely unhealthy as a food option.

If you really need to save time on food preparation, there are a number of alternatives that could be considered. Some of these include fresh fruit and vegetable outlets that sell fresh produce that's already been skinned and diced, literally ready to be added to the pot immediately with no preparation time at all. This goes for anything from frozen chopped mushrooms to crumbed onion rings. These may be slightly more expensive, but when you consider that you are paying for the fruit or vegetable by actual weight, without the skin and/or pips or seeds, you will realize that the costs are almost the same. Plus, there's something to be said for saving considerable amounts of time. If you are short on time and can afford the slightly more expensive option, they are worth it, as your time is precious.

These same food outlets sell meat and fish that's already filleted, prepared and ready to cook, making it easier than you could ever imagine to cook dinner from scratch. Almost anything you could imagine is available in a format that can be prepared fairly quickly with little to no fuss whatsoever. The benefit of going this route is that you can easily focus on big bouts of meal preparation to stock up your freezer or refrigerator with all the right food choices.

EATING OUT (WHILE INTUITIVE EATING)

Once you are in tune with both your body and your hunger, eating out should be no different than eating at home. If you know the restaurant or food establishment and have an idea of their portion sizes, it becomes easier to order a smaller portion, or order your side dishes to share with others at the table. Consider ordering any additional sauces on the side, rather than having them serve them together with the meal. That way, you have control over how much sauce you decide to pour over your meal.

Remember that even when eating out, you don't need to finish everything on your plate. You can ask for it to be put in a container to take it home with you (seeing as you are paying for the entire meal, after all).

If you know that you are going to indulge yourself by having dessert after your meal, skip the starter, or vice versa. Because you are going to a restaurant, it doesn't mean that you MUST eat a 3-course meal. Sometimes the best meal to have in a restaurant is a buffet as this allows you to be in full control over how much and what you choose to eat.

When you aren't in control of the menu because you've been invited to attend an event such as a wedding or bar mitzvah and there is going to be a set menu—once again, you do not need to eat everything put in front of you! This mantra is beginning to sound like a war cry at this stage, because it actually is. Learn to stop eating when you are satisfied. Place your knife and fork down and allow your plate to be removed. Your body will thank you for it throughout the night and the following day.

If you are celebrating a special occasion, remember that having that slice of cake, or dessert is not going to suddenly make you obese. It's healthy to live with a balanced relationship with food. That means that you allow yourself those little luxuries from time to time. Remember that when the 'diet' mentality says that you need to cut something out of your diet—it almost automatically appears on the list of things that you will crave consistently. The quote at the beginning of this chapter says it so succinctly. You need to be able to experience joy together with your food, rather than opting for a life that is bland, tasteless, and uninteresting.

10

SEEKING HELP AND FINDING A COMMUNITY

"The greatness of a community is most accurately measured by the compassionate action of its members."

— *CORETTA SCOTT KING*

Recovery from any form of addiction takes time, compassion and usually requires the support of others to be fully effective. Recovering from compulsive dieting is exactly the same. There is no difference to the challenges faced by anyone who is so used to doing things in a certain way to having to physically unlearn them and learning something completely different.

WHERE TO GO FROM HERE?

In this final chapter, we are going to look at where you can find the help and assistance you need while you transition from life as a compulsive dieter to living as someone who learns the art of intuitive eating. Mentally it can be challenging and exhausting to figure out whether you're going about things the right way. How can you tell whether the voice inside your head is actually your intuition speaking to you, or it is just yourself? And, if so, is there a difference?

QUESTIONS AND ANSWERS

So many questions that need to be answered on this intuitive eating journey. These are only a few of them:

- How do I know what foods I really like?
- How can I pick up on when I am feeling hungry rather than being ravenous due to emotional turmoil?
- How will I know if my body is receiving enough nutrition?
- What do I do if I'm hungry again in the middle of the night?

Because most of our lives are so busy and we do so much on the go—it's easy to skip some of these hunger cues. For the first while, you are going to need to pay close attention to what your body is saying to you, as and when it happens. It's like learning to tune into a specific radio frequency where the station is coming through loud and clear and the static or background noise is blocked out.

The answers to most of these questions are all actually common sense—even though we are often told that this is not so common! The single most important thing to learn from your experiments with intuitive eating is to judge how you feel while you are eating. Once you are able to do that, everything else will fall into place, and you will be able to enjoy the taste and texture of the food that you are eating, maybe for the first time in your life since you were very little. You will be able to slow down to appreciate the explosion of flavor happening in your mouth ... something that you've probably forgotten about because you're so used to grabbing a quick bite and eating on the run.

SLOWING LIFE DOWN

Life demands more and more of our time and there doesn't seem to be any way of stopping the fast pace or slowing it down. While we may not be able to change modern society or the pace of our work life, there are a few things that are actually under our control. As discussed in an earlier chapter, for example, we can slow life down by sitting together at a table for meals with our family. It builds relationships with our loved ones and gives us the ideal opportunity for practicing listening to what our intuition is telling us regarding the relationship that we have with our food. This relationship can either create a positive experience, where we've been able to take our time and enjoy what is in front of us, or it can result in a haphazard experience as we grab something on the go, not paying any attention to the taste, texture, our hunger level or whether we are satisfied.

We should make a real effort to eliminate multitasking while eating. This way we can enhance our eating experience. Focusing on our food allows us to become fully present in the moment and allows us to reconnect with our food preferences, as well as being in control of what we are eating and when.

HOW CAN THERAPY HELP?

Therapy can come to our aid in various forms when it comes to intuitive eating. If you're a recovering obsessive-compulsive dieter or chronic dieter, breaking the calorie counting habits of the past can be extremely difficult to do. For many, the mere thought of shopping without scanning each and every label to check ingredients can be daunting. It will often take a complete shift in mindset to change the self-defeating dieting belief system.

In many instances, this requires professional intervention by those who are qualified to offer this counsel and advice. Depending on the severity of the belief system surrounding body image you have acquired over the years, this may need to be referred to specialists who are able to deal with mental issues.

We are each different and therefore have the capacity and ability to face challenges and overcome them in different ways. For some, transitioning from being a compulsive dieter to an intuitive eater could be fairly smooth sailing. They may be able to read the supporting statistics and case studies and be able to accept that no diets are beneficial in the long term. On the other hand, others may need to attend multiple sessions of therapy or counseling sessions with dieticians, psychologists or even psychiatrists. It would all depend on how their self-image, self-esteem, or body image has been damaged. Those suffering from severe depression cannot and will not just be able to 'snap out of it' magically. It's important to be realistic and understand that this will take time.

ONLINE COMMUNITIES

There are many online communities that are there to support you in your journey towards intuitive eating. These could be found via online search engines such as Google or Bing; they're also often listed on platforms like Facebook and LinkedIn and if you make use of geo-tagging, you could probably find an actual in-person community in your region. Joining one of these groups may be an ideal way to start off your intuitive eating journey. Other members could help you by sharing some of what they've experienced with you. They may be able to share some advice that you could either use or discard if it's not really applicable to you. The upside of being able to communicate with those who have gone through it before you is that they are able to share some of the mistakes that they may have made in the past. This can help you avoid repeating these same mistakes yourself. Additionally, a community can offer a welcome reminder that you're not alone in this journey of self-acceptance and self-discovery. You may even make some new, non-dieting friends!

APPOINT A FRIEND

Share what you are doing with a close friend. Ask them to help you by holding you accountable. It needs to be someone that you can trust and that is strong enough to stand up to you and let you know when you're slipping, or out of line. Ways that they can hold you accountable is by setting specific goals with them. The journals that we've discussed throughout this book could be shared with them so they can monitor how you're doing. You could also schedule regular times to get together to discuss your progress. Don't procrastinate these meetings. Set them weekly for the first while, until you are feeling more confident and comfortable.

Once you've got the handle on it and you are comfortable with being able to hear your intuition telling you when you're hungry and when you've had enough, you can begin setting your meetings further apart. As much as possible, meet up in person. It's not as easy to hide what you're really experiencing when you're face to face.

ADDITIONAL RESOURCES

Since Evelyn Tribole and Elyse Resch first wrote *Intuitive Eating* in 1995, followers of this way of eating and living have popped up all over the world. Support groups are available, training is available, and research is ongoing even though it's been 25 years since this work was originally published. This should provide anyone wanting to kick the dieting habit for good a clear incentive that they won't be faced with doing it alone. Those who have managed to master it will be there right alongside you each step of the way.

AFTERWORD

Kicking the Diet Mindset has provided you with all the tools and information that you should ever need to never again be sucked into being duped into another diet fad, fashion, formula, or trends that makes promises it cannot keep. Instead of promising you miraculous weight loss overnight (the Nirvana of all things diet-related), intuitive eating allows you to completely change the way you think about food.

BAN THE BILLBOARDS

Intuitive eating is about taking control back and listening to your inner voice when it comes to eating rather than listening to what society is telling you instead. Society will always be in your face brandishing billboards, geo-tagging the websites you visit and spewing out images of the perfect look, the perfect image, the perfect body, shape, size, etc. Realize that all of these are just advertising gimmicks and tactics to get you to buy their products (in many instances, for you, this may be diet-related). Don't let them get into your head. Remember how many diets you've already tried and failed. That's been one of your main reasons for buying this book: you have been in search of a better way, a healthier way of doing things.

FOLLOWING THE FAMOUS

Following the lives of celebrities closely on Facebook, Instagram or Twitter can trigger strong emotions of negative body image or self-loathing because you don't look like them. What all of these advertising agencies, film companies and modeling agencies don't tell you is how much makeup is being applied, how much photoshopping takes place before things go to print or hit the marketplace. The pressure of conforming to the stereotypes that society demands we blindly accept as 'the norm', or the world requires, is too much to handle for most of us.

The secret to eliminating most of the pressure from how all of these images that you're surrounded with constantly is to get rid of as many of them as possible. It's learning to discover exactly who you are from the inside out—rather than from the outside in. The saying "beauty is only skin deep," by Sir Thomas Overbury (1613) is something that we should embrace and even write down and place in a prominent place in your home. This will remind you not to become preoccupied with your physical appearance to the point where it's leaving you miserable and depressed.

The solution to this problem is a simple one: hit the "unfollow" or "unlike" button on all of these accounts and begin looking for websites, forums, online communities and even celebrities that boost your self-image and your self-confidence. Sign up for these instead. There are loads of positive influencers for good out there who aren't going to make you empty promises at a high cost. Find the right accounts to follow and embrace the freedom that comes from finally understanding that looking 'perfect' isn't actually that important at all!

LEARN TO LOVE YOURSELF

Learning to love yourself as you are is one of the main aims of intuitive eating. It's retraining yourself to rediscover or form a new relationship with the food that you eat. Intuitive eating gives you back freedom from stressing about overindulging or binge eating. It skips past the guilt trip that potentially leads to anxiety and depression, which leads to further binge eating of comfort food ... and so the cycle continues.

Loving yourself promotes self-acceptance as you are right now, at this moment. It's not asking you to prove anything to anyone. You don't need to be a size 2 to be invited to this party of positive emotions. You can simply revert to reading through the list that you made in your journal about all the good things your body can do for you right now. As you become stronger, you will find that your lists will become even longer, allowing you to celebrate even more positive attributes. Celebrate each aspect of your body as it is right at this moment—recognizing what it's capable of and even what it can't do, and being at peace with that.

Come to terms with your body and learn to be okay with it. For many, this process is more like a journey that needs to be explored and discovered over time. Intuitive eating involves no magic lotions, potions, pills, or programs that are going to make you instantly lose weight that's making you feel bad about yourself. Instead, it breaks the chains of conventional diets that require calorie counting, weighing out portions or calculating how many calories you've managed to burn during the day in order to plan your evening meal. Intuitive eating sets you free from all of this stress and anxiety by going back to your roots, maybe for the first time in your life from when you were a toddler and your mother allowed you to eat whatever you wanted, leaving things on your plate and making your own decisions when it came to food. This is the point that you're trying to get back to.

PUT YOUR BODY BACK IN CHARGE

Intuitive eating puts your body back in the driving seat by teaching you to listen to when your body tells you you're hungry, rather than eating for the sake of eating. By listening to the same promptings that will let you know that you've had sufficient food to fuel your body, you'll begin to take back the control that's defined your relationship with food for most of your life. Allow yourself to make the decisions on what types of foods you want to eat. Choose those that you most enjoy and that make you feel happy. There's nothing worse than feeling that you have to drink only tomato and celery juice for a month in an attempt to shed a few pounds (not that intuitive eating is about losing weight).

AFTERWORD

LICENSE TO CHOOSE

Intuitive eating is not a license to go out there and binge-eat anything and everything, although this may be a learning curve that you need to go through to discover that there are consequences for not listening to when the body tells you it's full. Having to experience bloating and other side effects of overeating could allow you to begin to recognize what happens when you don't stop.

Intuitive eating is not a diet, it has not and never will be flaunted and promoted as a diet—not even going back to its original introduction in 1995 was it promoted as such. It's always been regarded as a way of finally ending the intimate war between yourself and food.

FORGIVING YOURSELF

Intuitive eating is about forgiving yourself for the way you look now. You may have been a victim of the dieting merry-go-round, on again and off again. Each time gaining slightly more weight than the time before. It's time to stop blaming your current weight issues on anything other than poor food relationships or choices. With intuitive eating, the buck needs to stop with you. You need to take full responsibility and ownership of your health, your body, and the food that you're choosing to put into your body.

Your old eating habits are now in the past. Clean the slate and make a decision to move on. Don't waste any valuable time by looking back at failed dieting attempts. If you begin this journey with intuitive eating, you need to be prepared to forgive yourself of all past choices and decisions and learn to let go.

CHOOSE HEALTH AND VITALITY

Intuitive eating is taking a holistic view of your health and vitality, especially when it relates to food. Accept and appreciate that you're not going to get the whole intuitive eating thing down immediately. It's going to be a process. It's going to be a journey. If you choose to share it with your family, friends, or other loved ones, it becomes more bearable because they will hold you accountable. Having to check in with someone to discuss how it's going makes it more difficult to return to old ways.

Being healthier through making better food choices will always influence and impact other areas of your life. It's not about losing weight, but rather about choosing a lifestyle that's going to lead to improved health and happiness.

OLD HABITS DIE HARD

Be patient with yourself when you catch yourself still counting calories in a store or reading food labels. Remind yourself that you no longer need to do that. Allow yourself the freedom to enjoy treats occasionally. Remember that one slice of cake or pizza is not going to destroy your lifestyle. Remind yourself over and over again that intuitive eating is a lifestyle rather than a diet. Give yourself the time that you need to make the changes in your eating patterns. Although this may be difficult to do at first, as you practice listening and watching for the hunger cues that your body provides you with, you will realize when you need to eat and when to set your knife and fork down.

ENJOY YOUR MEALS

Take your time over meals, reintroduce old traditions of eating at a dinner table once more. Celebrate the food that's in front of you, savoring it by eating more slowly than you normally would if you were multi-tasking. If you're in the workplace, make a point of not eating at your desk while you're working. Instead, get up and eat your meal in a canteen, on a park bench or somewhere away from the office.

Allowing yourself to be distracted while eating could often allow for overeating to occur. Because your focus is divided between your meal and your work, your phone, or the tv, it becomes impossible to hear the body's cues that are telling you that you have had enough.

Chew your food thoroughly and take smaller bite sizes versus shoveling everything down in a matter of seconds. Not only will this give you time to savor the food in front of you, but you'll enjoy the meal more. Greater appreciation for the taste of the food leads to feeling satisfied. This is the point where you need to set your knife and fork down.

ALLOW YOU TO BE YOU

The most important key to intuitive eating is to allow yourself to be who you truly are. It's falling in love with yourself and accepting your body the way that it is right now. While we've spoken about keeping journals for your food journey and activities, you could either add to it, or you can do this by beginning and keeping a new journal of all the things you're grateful for that your body can do, as it is—right now!

It's replacing feelings of self-loathing with feelings of self-care and learning to be kinder and gentler towards yourself. Self-love is centered on accepting that we are all unique and have something to contribute to the world. Discovering exactly what this is may take time, effort, and some deep soul-searching. It's getting to know exactly who you are and loving yourself for it. In a world that wants you to think you're not enough (so that people can sell you things), self-love is a revolutionary act. Be brave!

MOVING FORWARD

Your personal journey towards self-discovery through intuitive eating is just one step away. All that it needs from you is a desire to begin... Remember that there are people out there who have walked this path before you. There are support groups and online communities just waiting for you to reach out and join them.

All that it's going to take on your part is a willingness to walk away from the dieting mentality forever and look at discovering exactly who you are. You are strong enough—you've got this!

REFERENCES

(2017). Exercise 'keeps the mind sharp' in over-50s, study finds. – BBC News. https://www.bbc.com/news/health-39693462

10 Principles of Intuitive Eating. (n.d.). https://www.intuitiveeating.org/10-principles-of-intuitive-eating/

10 Steps to Positive Body Image. (n.d.). https://www.nationaleatingdisorders.org/learn/general-information/ten-steps

Barghouty, L. (2020). What Intuitive Eating Can & Can't Do, According To Experts. https://www.bustle.com/p/what-intuitive-eating-can-cant-do-according-to-experts-21814401

Barraclough, E. L., Hay-Smith, E. J. C., Boucher, S. E., Tylka, T. L., Howarth, C. C., (2019). Learning to eat intuitively: A qualitative exploration of the experience of mid-age women. https://www.ncbi.nlm.nih.gov/pmc/articles/PMC6360478

Barker, M. (2019). Intuitive eating: a 'diet' that actually makes sense. https://theconversation.com/intuitive-eating-a-diet-that-actually-makes-sense-112800

Bendsen, N. T., et al. (2013). Is Beer Consumption Related to Measures of Abdominal and General Obesity? A Systematic Review and Meta-Analysis - PubMed. https://pubmed.ncbi.nlm.nih.gov/23356635/

Benito-Corchon, S., Bes-Rastollo, M. (2014). Glycemic load, glycemic index, bread and incidence of overweight/obesity in a Mediterranean cohort: the SUN project. BMC Public Health. doi:10.1186/1471-2458-14-1091

Benshosan, A. (2018). The Reason Most Americans Diet Isn't Weight Loss—It's This. https://www.eatthis.com/reason-people-go-diet/

Body Image. (n.d.). https://www.nationaleatingdisorders.org/body-image-0

Brazier, Y. (2017). Body image: What is it and how can I improve it? https://www.medicalnewstoday.com/articles/249190

Bruce, L. J., Ricciardelli, L. A. (2016). A systematic review of the psychosocial correlates of intuitive eating among adult women. https://www.sciencedirect.com/science/article/abs/pii/S0195666315300635

Cash, T. F., Smolak, L. (2011). Body Image, Second Edition: A Handbook of Science, Practice, and Prevention. New York: Guilford Press.

Dillon, J. D. (n.d.). The Love Food Podcast. https://podcasts.apple.com/us/podcast/the-love-food-podcast/id1076673018

Disordered Eating & Dieting. (n.d.). https://www.nedc.com.au/eating-disorders/eating-disorders-explained/disordered-eating-and-dieting/

Dodier, S. (2019). Intuitive Eating Made Simple: A Step-by-Step Guide. https://thriveglobal.com/stories/intuitive-eating-made-simple-a-step-by-step-guide/

Downs, M. (n.d.). Why Do We Keep Falling for Fad Diets? https://www.webmd.com/diet/features/why-do-we-keep-falling-for-fad-diets

Flores, A. (2018). What Does Intuitive Eating Mean? https://www.nationaleatingdisorders.org/blog/what-does-intuitive-eating-mean

Frey, M. (2019). How to Start a Workout Routine If You're Overweight. https://www.verywellfit.com/best-workouts-if-youre-overweight-3495993

Gavin, M. L. (n d.). The Deal With Diets (for Teens) – Nemours KidsHealth. https://kidshealth.org/en/teens/dieting.html

Gingell, S. (2018). How Your Mental Health Reaps the Benefits of Exercise: New research shows why physical exercise is essential to mental health. https://www.psychologytoday.com/za/blog/what-works-and-why/201803/how-your-mental-health-reaps-the-benefits-exercise

Harrison, C. (n.d.) Podcast - Christy Harrison - Intuitive Eating Dietician, Anti-Diet Author, & Health at Every Size Advocate - Food Psych Programs. https://christyharrison.com/foodpsych

Hartley, R. (2015). Three Exercises for Newbie Intuitive Eaters. https://www.rachaelhartleynutrition.com/blog/2015/06/exercises-for-new-intuitive-eaters

Heart Matters Magazine. 10 Principles of intuitive eating. (n.d.). https://www.bhf.org.uk/informationsupport/heart-matters-magazine/nutrition/weight/intuitive-eating/10-principles-of-intuitive-eating

Hunt, T. (2019). Intuitive Eating Sounds Great, But What If I Still Want To Lose Weight? https://tailoredcoachingmethod.com/intuitive-eating/

Imma Eat That. (n.d.). https://immaeatthat.com/

Intuitive Eating Quotes by Evelyn Tribole. (n.d.) https://www.goodreads.com/work/quotes/228458-intuitive-eating-a-revolutionary-program-that-works

Jennings, K. (2019). A Quick Guide to Intuitive Eating. https://www.healthline.com/nutrition/quick-guide-intuitive-eating

John Hopkins Medicine. (n.d.). Exercising for Better Sleep https://www.hopkinsmedicine.org/health/wellness-and-prevention/exercising-for-better-sleep

Johnson, B. (2012). Mind - Body - Nutrition: Nutritional psychologist Marc David explains why our mental and emotional responses to food matter far more than we realize. https://experiencelife.com/article/mind-body-nutrition/

Jones, J. (2019). So You Want to Try Intuitive Eating, but If You're Being Honest, You Still Want to Watch Your Weight. What to Do? https://www.self.com/story/intuitive-eating-and-weight-loss

Karges, C. (n.d.). Intuitive Eating Principles as a Family. https://www.eatingdisorderhope.com/blog/learning-intuitive-eating-principles-as-a-family

Landsverk, G. (2020). 'Intuitive eating' is on the rise, and experts say it's because people are fed up with diet culture. https://www.insider.com/what-is-intuitive-eating-does-it-work-2020-1

Leal, D. (2020). Improve Your Health With Intuitive Eating: Say "No" to Diets and "Yes" to a Healthy Relationship With Food. https://www.verywellfit.com/overview-of-intuitive-eating-4178361

London, J. (2019). What Is Intuitive Eating? How to Eat Better Without Dieting, According to Nutritionists: Forget calorie counting and food restricting—this philosophy is all about listening to your body. https://www.goodhousekeeping.com/health/diet-nutrition/a26324845/intuitive-eating/

Mandl, E. (2019). Binge Eating Disorder: Symptoms, Causes, and Asking for Help. https://www.healthline.com/nutrition/binge-eating-disorder

Muhlheim, L. (2020). How Can Intuitive Eating Help My Eating Disorder? https://www.verywellmind.com/intuitive-eating-can-help-disordered-eating-4796957

Nutrition Matters Podcast | Positive Nutrition. (n.d.). https://www.positive-nutrition.com/podcast

Positive Body Image. (n.d.). https://www.skillsyouneed.com/ps/positive-body-image.html

Quotes About The Power of Community. (n.d.). https://www.ellevatenetwork.com/articles/8538-quotes-about-the-power-of-community

Rollin, J. (2015). 3 Reasons You Should Never Go on a Diet: Research shows a surprising percentage of us simply can't keep it off long-term. https://www.psychologytoday.com/us/blog/mindful-musings/201510/3-reasons-you-should-never-go-diet

Rumsey, A. (2017). How to Get Started with Intuitive Eating. https://alissarumsey.com/intuitive-eating/how-to-start-intuitive-eating/

Rumsey, A. (2017). Ask Yourself This Before (and

After) You Eat. https://alissarumsey.com/nutrition/hunger-fullness-scale/

Rumsey, A. (2019). How to Practice Intuitive Movement. https://alissarumsey.com/fitness/intuitive-exercise-tips/

Rumsey, A. (2019). What is Intuitive Eating? https://www.alissarumsey.com/intuitive-eating/what-is-intuitive-eating/

Sauer, M., Olsen, N. (2018). 7 Things I Learned During My First Week of Intuitive Eating. https://www.healthline.com/health/my-first-week-of-intuitive-eating

Schaefer, J. T., Magnuson, A. B. (2014). A Review of Interventions that Promote Eating by Internal Cues | Science Direct https://www.sciencedirect.com/science/article/abs/pii/S2212267213018960

Stenovec, L. (n.d.). The Embodied & Well mom show. https://www.intuitiveeatingmoms.com/podcast-2/

The Foodie Dietitian Blog by Kara Lydon, RD | Kara Lydon (n.d.). https://karalydon.com/blog

The Phrase Finder: The meaning and origin of the expression: Beauty is only skin deep. (n.d.). https://www.phrases.org.uk/meanings/59200.html

The Real Life RD, (n.d.). https://www.thereallife-rd.com

Timmons, J., Pletcher, P. (2016). How Sedentary Obese People Can Ease Into Regular Exercise. https://www.healthline.com/health/fitness-exercise/exercise-for-obese-people

To thine own self be true – eNotes Shakespeare Quotes. (n.d.). https://www.enotes.com/shakespeare-quotes/thine-own-self-true

Tribole, E. (n.d.). Intuitive Eating Resources.

https://www.evelyntribole.com/resources/intuitive-eating-resources/

Van Dyke, N., Drinkwater, E. J., (2014). Relationships between intuitive eating and health indicators: literature review. – PubMed. https://www.ncbi.nlm.nih.gov/pubmed/23962472

www.ingramcontent.com/pod-product-compliance
Lightning Source LLC
Chambersburg PA
CBHW020258030426
42336CB00010B/820